Complete Dental Bleaching

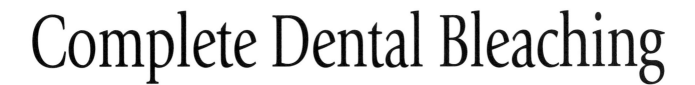

Complete Dental Bleaching

Ronald E. Goldstein, DDS

Clinical Professor of Oral Rehabilitation
School of Dentistry
Medical College of Georgia
Augusta, Georgia

Adjunct Clinical Professor of Prosthodontics
Goldman School of Graduate Dentistry
Boston University
Boston, Massachusetts

Visiting Professor of Oral and Maxillofacial
Imaging and Continuing Education
School of Dentistry
University of Southern California
Los Angeles, California

Adjunct Professor of Restorative Dentistry
University of Texas Health Science Center
San Antonio, Texas

David A. Garber, BDS, DMD

Clinical Professor of Periodontics
School of Dentistry
Medical College of Georgia
Augusta, Georgia

Clinical Professor of Oral Rehabilitation
School of Dentistry
Medical College of Georgia
Augusta, Georgia

quintessence books

Quintessence Publishing Co, Inc
Chicago, Berlin, London, Tokyo, São Paulo, Moscow, Prague, Warsaw

Library of Congress Cataloging-in-Publication Data

Goldstein, Ronald E.
    Complete dental bleaching/Ronald E. Goldstein, David A. Garber.
           p.   cm.
    Includes bibliographical references and index.
    ISBN 0-86715-290-7
    1. Teeth—Bleaching. I. Garber, David A. II. Title
    [DNLM: 1. Tooth Bleaching. 2. Tooth Discoloration—therapy. WU 166 G624c 1995
    RK320.B55G65 1995
  617.6'34—dc20
  DNLM/DLC
  for Library of Congress   95-14260
                                           CIP

© 1995 by Quintessence Publishing Co, Inc
All rights reserved.

Editor: Adam Haus
Designer: Jennifer Sabella
Printed by Everbest Printing, Hong Kong.

Contents

Contributors

Howard Frysh, BDS, DDS
Associate Professor
College of Dentistry
Baylor University
Dallas, Texas

Van B. Haywood, DMD
Associate Professor
Department of Oral Rehabilitation
School of Dentistry
Medical College of Georgia
Augusta, Georgia

Harald O. Heymann, DDS, MEd
Chair, Department of Operative Dentistry
School of Dentistry
University of North Carolina
Charlotte, North Carolina

David R. Steiner, DDS, MSD
Clinical Associate Professor
Department of Endodontics
School of Dentistry
University of Washington
Seattle, Washington

John D. West, DDS, MSD
Clinical Associate Professor
Department of Endodontics
School of Dentistry
University of Washington
Seattle, Washington

Preface

Few dental treatments have been more successful in the past decade than bleaching teeth. Both in-office and at-home treatments have captured the attention of the lay public throughout the world. People can now have more control than ever over the appearance and coloration of their teeth and, in most cases, even play a role in obtaining their desired result.

Since 1976, when the first chapter on tooth bleaching appeared in an esthetic dentistry textbook (Goldstein, *Esthetics in Dentistry*), techniques and results have improved dramatically. Not only has the public embraced the concept, but dentists have integrated it as a routine, rapid, and conservative part of their esthetic armamentarium.

This text shows just how much the science of tooth bleaching has become part of the esthetic dental arena. Dr Howard Frysh's chapter on the chemistry of bleaching provides the scientific information as to how and why tooth bleaching is so effective. Drs Haywood and Heymann complement the in-office bleaching chapter with detailed attention to nightguard vital bleaching, just as Drs Steiner and West provide an important new look at bleaching the pulpless tooth. The final chapter integrates all of the various esthetic dental modalities and demonstrates how bleaching can be an integral part of most interdisciplinary treatment plans. We hope that this book will encourage appropriate use of bleaching in your practice of esthetic dentistry.

Acknowledgments

No text we write would be complete without the constant help we receive from our office secretaries, Margie Smith, Cynthia Clement, and Candace Paetzhold. The administrative and research assistance of Susan Hodgson, coupled with her writing skills, improved the final version of the text.

We would like to acknowledge the technical photographic advice and help received from Mr Howard Golden and Mr John Johnny of the Minolta Corporation. Most of the photographs and slides were made using the Minolta 7000 or 7XI with a 100-mm macro lens and the 1200 AF electronic flash unit.

Most of the combined-therapy cases were the work of our master ceramist, Pinhas Adar, an integral part of our esthetic team.

Finally, we are ever mindful of the tremendous sacrifice our families make in allowing us to take extra time away from them to be able to produce a text such as this one. So, to Judy, Barbara, Karen, Jennifer, and Michael we say thank you for all your love and support.

A New Role for Restorative Dentistry

Does Bleaching Belong in My Practice?

The last three decades have witnessed immense changes in dentistry, beginning with the profession's dramatic and unprecedented success in the reduction of caries and periodontal disease. The subsequent decline in what had been the primary activities in dentistry caused many dentists to reexamine and redefine their roles in meeting the dental needs of their patients. Perhaps the single most significant change was contemporary dentistry's new emphasis on esthetics. This was a direct result of dentists' ability to bond predictably to teeth, allowing patients to keep sound tooth structure while improving their looks.

Attractive teeth have always been the typical patient's primary concern. In the past, dentists were often dismayed by a patient's disappointment in a "perfect restoration," painstakingly crafted of the finest gold or other material, with minimized enamel reduction and long-lasting preservation of function. The patient, of course, had hoped the restoration would mimic the appearance of the original teeth. Today, by taking full advantage of new materials and techniques, dentists can often meet or even exceed such expectations.

What most people really want, however, are teeth that make them look younger, healthier, and more attractive. Thirty years ago, patients considered dentists both allies in the prevention of dental problems and friendly repair professionals when such problems inevitably occurred. Today, dentists are increasingly becoming the professionals to whom people turn first for advice and assistance on improving their appearance. The increase of adult orthodontics is one measure of this trend. The sharp rise in the acceptance and demand for treatments of otherwise healthy teeth to make them brighter and whiter is an even better measure.

The question is no longer whether or not to add bleaching to your practice. To provide the services increasingly expected by your patients and provided by your colleagues, you have to provide bleaching.

Bleaching is now the single most common esthetic treatment for adults. We estimate that more than a million people have had teeth bleached by dentists, while perhaps millions more have tried their own hand at bleaching with over-the-counter products. The popularity of bleaching is easily understood. For the appropriate patient, with careful diagnosis, case selection, treatment planning, and attention to technique, bleaching is the simplest, least invasive, least expensive means available to lighten discolored teeth and diminish or eliminate many stains in both vital and pulpless teeth. Once considered the province of a few pioneering specialists in esthetic dentistry, bleaching has now moved into the mainstream of restorative dentistry. A growing number of your patients are probably asking you what bleaching can do for them now. The question is no longer whether or not to add bleaching to your practice. To provide the services increasingly expected by your patients and provided by your colleagues, you have to provide bleaching.

But bleaching is not a simple yes-or-no treatment option, especially as a larger number and wider range of patients expect and ask for brighter teeth. Patients interested in bleaching range from children to senior citizens; from the well-to-do to those who must keep costs at the bare minimum; from the person with a single deeply discolored pulpless tooth to one with a smile yellowed by years of staining, various diseases, systemic medication intake, or simply aging. More significantly, some patients' only problem is tooth discoloration, while others have periodontal problems, tooth malalignment, and caries requiring preliminary attention.

For a few patients, one or two in-office bleaching sessions will produce results that seem almost miraculous. For a few patients—and it's essential to recognize which few—bleaching may never be a safe or appropriate therapy. But for the majority of patients seeking more attractive smiles, bleaching holds out a varying amount of promise for improvement, especially when used as an adjunct to other cosmetic procedures. In combination with other esthetic procedures, such as microabrasion, lightening a stained tooth before veneering, or crowning to improve the color of adjacent teeth, bleaching expands the scope of esthetic dentistry. In the 1980s and 1990s, new partnerships and referral patterns have given bleaching a new role as an adjunct to orthodontics, orthognathic surgery, endodontics, and restorative dental treatments, as well as to treatments in dermatology, plastic and reconstructive surgery, and other fields. In fact, an increasing number of dentists and other health professionals concerned with esthetics are asking all patients if they are satisfied with the color of their teeth. The appropriate questions for today's dentist, therefore, are how best to incorporate various methods and materials of bleaching into total treatment plans and how best to work with a team of dental and other professionals to achieve the patient's objectives. These are the primary questions this book is designed to answer.

> *The appropriate questions for today's dentist, therefore, are how best to incorporate various methods and materials of bleaching into total treatment plans and how best to work with a team of dental and other professionals to achieve the patient's objectives.*

What Are the Major Causes of Discoloration?

Superficial Changes Affecting Only the Enamel Surface

These usually are caused by habitual use of highly colored foods or beverages such as tea, coffee, and cola, all of which can cause tenacious brown to black discolorations. Nicotine is another cause of dark surface stains. Smoking tobacco cigarettes, cigars, or pipes produces a yellowish brown to black discoloration, usually in the cervical portion of the teeth and primarily on the lingual surfaces, while smoking marijuana may produce sharply delineated rings around the cervical portion of the teeth adjacent to the gingival margins. Chewing tobacco frequently penetrates microcracks in the enamel to produce an even darker stain, in addition to the soft tissue problems often found in users. All of these surface stains are highly amenable to bleaching, although stains are more difficult to remove from pits, fissures, grooves, or enamel defects. If microcracks have allowed the stain to permeate the tooth, bleaching may not be as appropriate or effective as some of the newer conservative restorative treatments (Figs 1-1a and 1-1b).

Discoloration of the Tooth Structure

Teeth can become stained and discolored, sometimes before they even erupt (Figs 1-2a and 1-2b), when the tooth structure itself is altered by a discoloring agent. This happens in a variety of ways:

Medication Given Systemically, Especially During Tooth Formation

Dentists first recognized the devastating effect some medications could have on tooth formation in the late 1950s, when large numbers of young people began displaying yellow, brown, or gray stains caused by the antibiotic tetracycline.[1] The first certain identification was reported in a study of cystic fibrosis patients, for whom tetracycline was (and unfortunately remains) one of the most effective treatments for control of secondary infection of the respiratory system. The severity of the stains and specific color depend on the type of tetracycline administered (more than 2,000 variants have been patented), the duration of use, and the stage of tooth formation at the time of use.

In fact, tetracycline provided dentists much insight into the mechanism by which medications could result in intrinsic stains. Teeth are most susceptible to tetracycline discoloration during formation, beginning with the second trimester in utero and

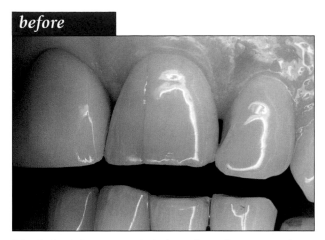

Fig 1-1a This patient's habit of smoking several packs of cigarettes per day stained the teeth, making the microcracks even more prominent, as typified in the left central incisor.

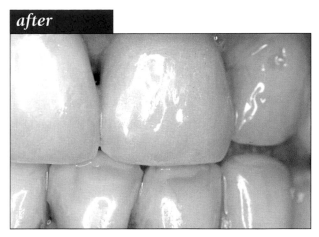

Fig 1-1b Although the teeth were bleached and the patient's smoking habit was reversed, a ceramic alternative was chosen to improve the left central incisor.

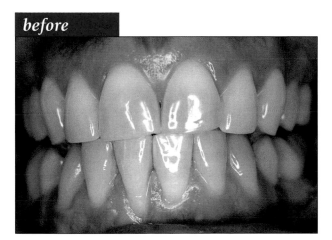

Fig 1-2a High fever or certain medications can cause individual tooth defects or tooth discoloration, depending upon occurrence or administration. Note dark staining on two-thirds of the labial surface of this patient's central incisors.

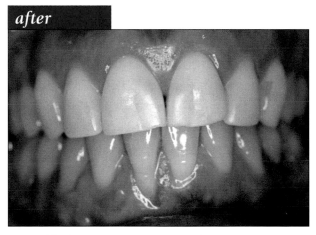

Fig 1-2b A combination of in-office and matrix home bleaching was successful not only in eliminating the stain but also in lightening the patient's teeth.

examination of the affected teeth will show a hypomineralized, porous subsurface enamel and a well-mineralized surface layer. This enamel hypoplasia is termed *endemic enamel fluorosis* or "mottled enamel." The premolar teeth are the most commonly affected, followed by second molars, maxillary incisors, canines and first molars, and mandibular incisors. Where fluoride concentration is very high, primary teeth may also be affected.

Affected teeth usually have glazed surfaces and may be paper white, with areas of yellow, brown, or even black shading in any location on the teeth. Stains may range from a simple brown diffuse pigmentation on a smooth enamel surface (Figs 1-4a and 1-4b) to opaque fluorosis, with flat gray or white flecks or larger white or opaque spots visible on the enamel surface.

Bleaching can be an effective treatment modality for this type of discoloration. If the mottling is serious enough, the enamel may be chalky, without the glaze and luster of a normal tooth. If staining is accompanied by pitting and other surface defects, bleaching is best viewed as a useful adjunctive treatment preceding bonding or veneering. If fluorosis has caused severe loss of enamel, bleaching should not be used at all.

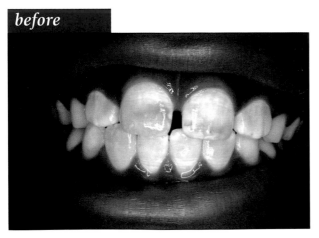

Fig 1-4a Fluorosis is the cause of this brown pigmentation.

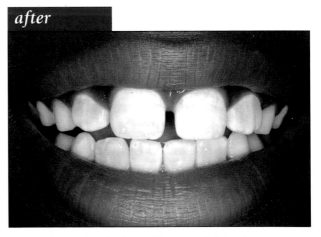

Fig 1-4b Individual in-office tooth bleaching was effective in eliminating the stain and producing a more pleasing smile.

Stain From Systemic Conditions

Although there are a number of genetic conditions or childhood illnesses that cause discoloration of the teeth, most are rare and infrequently seen. However, for those conditions in which discoloration results from a pigment infusion of the dentin during development, bleaching can be quite effective. These conditions include the bluish-green or brown primary teeth that result from postnatal dentin staining by bilirubin in children who suffered severe jaundice as infants; the characteristically brownish teeth caused by destruction of an excessive number of blood-cell erythrocytes in erythroblastosis fetalis, a result of Rh-factor incompatibility between mother and fetus; and the purplish-brown teeth of persons with porphyria, a rare condition that causes an excess production of pigment.

> *Bleaching is usually a less appropriate treatment than bonding or crowning when illness has caused discoloration of the teeth by interfering with the normal matrix formation or calcification of the enamel.*

Bleaching is usually a less appropriate treatment than bonding or crowning when illness has caused discoloration of the teeth by interfering with the normal matrix formation or calcification of the enamel. Hypoplasia or hypocalcification can occur with genetic conditions like amelogenesis imperfecta and clefting of the lip and palate or with acquired illnesses such as cerebral palsy, serious renal damage, and severe allergies. Brain, neurological, and other traumatic injuries also can interfere with the normal development of the enamel. Deficiencies of vitamins C and D and of calcium and phosphorous during enamel's formative period can cause hypoplasia.

Stain From Dental Conditions or Treatments

Dental caries are a primary cause of pigmentation, appearing as either an opaque white halo or a gray cast. An even deeper brown to black discoloration can result from bacterial degradation of food debris in areas of tooth decay. Tooth-colored restorations such as acrylics, glass ionomers, or composites can cause teeth to look grayer and discolored as the restoration ages and degrades

(Figs 1-5a and 1-5b). Metal restorations, even silver amalgams and gold inlays, can reflect discoloration through the enamel, a problem that may become more evident with the thinning and translucency of enamel that occurs with aging (Fig 1-6). Bleaching may not be necessary once the proper repair or replacement of these restorations takes place.

A more difficult discoloration occurs when oils, iodines, nitrates, root-canal sealers, pins, and other materials used in dental restoration have penetrated the dentinal tubules. The length of time the substance has penetrated the tubules will determine the amount of residual discoloration and, consequently, the success of bleaching.

Tooth Color Changes Due to Aging

Changes in tooth color, as well as tooth form and texture, almost inevitably accompany aging. Most newly formed teeth have thick, even enamel which modifies the base color of the underlying dentin.[10] That bright, milky white appearance seems to be the ideal in today's society. Unfortunately, all of the numerous genetic, environmental, medical, and dental causes described above move teeth further away from that ideal, and aging intensifies all of their effects. Food and drink have a cumulative staining effect, and these and other stains become even more visible in the older patient because of the inevitable cracking and other changes on the enamel surface of the tooth, within its crystalline structure, and in the underlying dentin. Furthermore, amalgams and other restorations placed years ago inevitably degrade over time, causing further staining.

Were these environmental assaults not problem enough, aging usually brings a thinning of the enamel, which may cause the facial surface of the tooth to appear flat with a progressive shift in color due to a loss of the translucent enamel layer. At the same time as the enamel begins to thin, secondary dentin formation, a natural tooth protective mechanism in the dentin and pulp, further exacerbates the problem. The combination of less enamel and more darkened, opaque dentin creates an older-looking tooth. Unless the enamel is very badly worn, however, bleaching can be an effective treatment for many of the discolorations seen in older patients. As Chapter 3 explains, bleaching is particularly appealing for many patients because of the minimal chair time, expense, and potential for postoperative sensitivity due to recession of the pulp (Figs 1-7a and 1-7b).

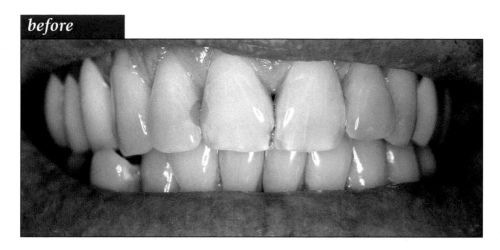

Fig 1-5a Discolored composites accentuated unattractive yellowed teeth.

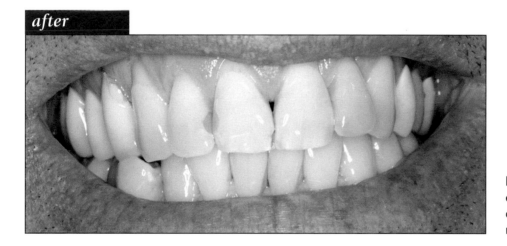

Fig 1-5b Bleaching lightened the teeth but did not change the color of the restorations.

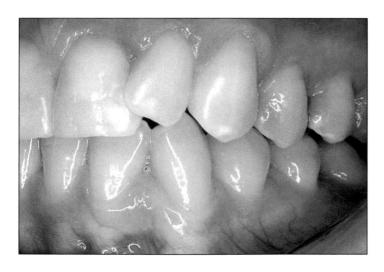

Fig 1-6 This patient wanted a lighter look to her smile and objected to the discoloration caused by her old amalgams in the premolar area. Bleaching alone has improved this stain; however, total resolution will only be accomplished by replacement of the old amalgams.

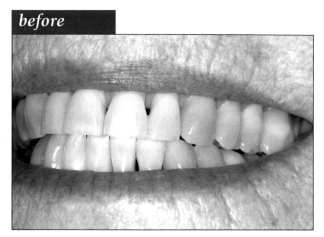

Fig 1-7a These discolored teeth are a sign of an aging smile. Bleaching could help provide a more youthful look.

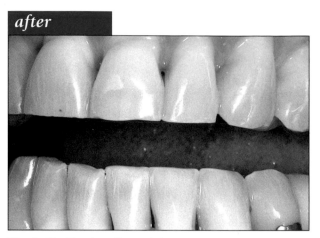

Fig 1-7b Teeth yellowed due to age can be excellent candidates for both in-office or matrix bleaching.

Bleaching: An Evolving History

Bleaching is not new! The earliest efforts to lighten teeth through bleaching took place more than a century ago, with bleaching agents painted directly on the tooth surface or packed inside a nonvital tooth. The earliest agent reportedly used was oxalic acid, described by Chappel in 1877.[11] Following experiments with various forms of chlorine, Harlan described in 1884 what is believed to be the first use of hydrogen peroxide, which he called hydrogen dioxide.[11]

Although many of the mechanisms by which bleaching removes discoloration are not yet fully understood (see Chapter 2 for an explanation of bleaching chemistry), the basic process involves oxidation, in which the bleaching agent enters the enamel/ dentin of the discolored tooth and releases the molecules containing the discoloration. How well it works depends upon the cause of the stain; where, how deeply, and how long the stain has permeated the structure of the tooth; and how well the bleaching agent can permeate to the source of the discoloration and remain there long enough to release deep stains. If the stains are on the surface or subsurface of the tooth, the process is fairly simple. The addition of mild etching to remove surface organic material appears to enhance this process by cleaning the teeth and perhaps by exposing slightly deeper areas of enamel to the bleach. But hydrogen peroxide alone can permeate through the surface of the tooth to reach stained enamel and dentin and release discoloration that has penetrated the tooth's inner structure.

Once hydrogen peroxide was established as the most effective bleaching agent, dentists turned their attention to finding ways to facilitate its absorption and penetration to speed the oxidation process. Early efforts included use of electric current and ultraviolet light.[11] In 1918, Abbot discovered what remains the basic combination used today: a high-intensity light that produces a rapid rise in the temperature of the hydrogen peroxide to accelerate the chemical process of bleaching.[12] Since then, the history of bleaching has been one of continuous improvement in the effectiveness and ease of use of bleaching agents, heat and light catalyst devices, and alternative methods, the most contemporary of which are described throughout this book.

Bleaching nonvital or pulpless teeth changed less rapidly. The first reported instance of bleaching nonvital teeth was in 1895, when a dentist named Garretson applied chloride to the tooth surface. The results were not inspiring, and there were few followers. But in 1958 Pearson realized the dentist could take advantage of the nonvital tooth's lack of a pulp. He packed the same hydrogen peroxide agent being used for bleaching of vital teeth, Superoxol, in the pulp chamber for 3 days.[13] By the late 1960s the standard method was established by Nutting and Poe, who sealed a mixture of 30% hydrogen peroxide and sodium perborate in the pulp chamber for up to a week.[14] Chapter 6 describes in detail the continuing improvements in bleaching of the nonvital tooth.

More recently, we have seen introduction of an alternative method to facilitate absorption of the bleaching agent by applying a weaker bleaching solution to the teeth for longer periods, usually by placing it in a retainer-like matrix worn by the patient for extended periods. Chapter 5 covers the rationale, indications, and step-by-step methodology for this immensely popular approach to whiter teeth.

Bleaching is now moving into a new phase of development. In its first phase at the turn of the century, bleaching teeth was a rather provocative, experimental modality. In its second phase, despite the fact that dentists recognized its effectiveness and safety in the middle of this century, bleaching was usually seen as a last-ditch effort to correct a particularly disfiguring discoloration, performed on highly selected patients by a few pioneering dentists interested in esthetic dentistry. Most general dentists used more familiar restorative methods, such as crowns and the newer restorative materials then available. Their hesitancy began to change somewhat in the 1970s with the dramatic results obtained for thousands of children with tetracycline staining or with surface discolorations from fluorosis. In its third phase, bleaching became more acceptable as an effective and safe in-office treatment for a wider spectrum of cases, but it still seemed to remain the province of the specialist and relatively few general dentists. Today, in the fourth and doubtless not yet the final stage, in-office and matrix bleaching are household words, and most dentists consider themselves esthetic dentists. The development of accessible computer imaging for the dental practice continues to enhance patient understanding, expectation, and satisfaction with innovative esthetic techniques and further improves the collaborations between dental and other specialists involved in esthetic enhancements.

Throughout this evolution, there have been two consistent questions in the research that accompanied clinical development:

1.   How well does bleaching work?

As presented in this chapter, the efficacy of bleaching depends on many factors, ranging from the type of stain, through the condition of teeth, to patient compliance during and following treatment. Goldstein[9] and Jordan and Boksman[4] estimate that vital bleaching is effective in as many as three-fourths of selected cases. There is also concern with long-term effectiveness, since for most patients there is an immediate loss of the bleaching effect in the first weeks following treatment and virtually all patients need retreatment within 3 years for a continuing optimal effect. Chapter 7 describes this work in more detail.

2.   How safe is it?

The use of any of the current bleaching agents is not totally without risk, and care must be taken in their storage, application, and monitoring.

As will be shown, protecting the eyes, skin, and soft tissue of the patient (as well as the dental team) from potential damaging effects of either heat, light, or the bleaching agent itself has always been an essential part of the in-office treatment process. The lack of anesthesia during in-office bleaching assures that any microscopic leak in the rubber dam would be noticed and corrected immediately.

Most of the earlier studies of in-office bleaching during the late 1970s and 1980s focused on possible deleterious damage to the pulp in vital teeth. It has been known for more than 40 years that substances can penetrate through enamel and dentin into the pulp. The low molecular weight of hydrogen peroxide and its capability to denature proteins probably enhances its ability to penetrate teeth.[13] Numerous studies of canine, bovine, and human teeth have looked at various solutions of hydrogen peroxide, heat applications, and combinations of the two in potential damage.[12,15-24] The earliest results were positive but cautionary, demonstrating that a technique of low heat application of approximately 98° to 140°F, using a 30% to 35% hydrogen peroxide solution, can sometimes cause some low-grade reversible pulpal inflammation and possible hard tooth structure damage. These findings have encouraged the establishment of current protocols involving shorter bleach time and restricted heat use.

> *Safety issues may be more pressing when bleaching pulpless teeth.*

As Sakaguchi and Hampel point out,[23] there have been only a few reports of side-effects resulting from bleaching therapy of vital teeth. These included mild inflammatory responses in teeth treated with heat and hydrogen peroxide, while the controlled use of saline and heat or hydrogen peroxide without heat did not cause a significant number of inflammatory responses.[23]

Safety issues may be more pressing when bleaching pulpless teeth. Although bleaching of pulpless teeth offers the most dramatic changes in appearance, it offers the greatest potential hazard; . . . cervical resorption of the tooth.[25] Chapter 6 describes the choices of technique, placement of the bleaching agent within the tooth, and bleaching materials that can make this as safe as most other commonly used dental treatments.

Finally, the rapid increase in home bleaching has caused an increased concern for safety. Chapter 5 describes the current findings in more detail, but reports suggest that, in general, the short-term safety and efficiency for hydrogen peroxide systems appear high.[26] Lower concentrations of hydrogen peroxide have been found to be less likely to cause oral irritation.

Advantages of Bleaching Used Alone

For most patients, the preeminent advantage of bleaching is its relatively low cost. A second advantage that leads many patients to inquire about bleaching is the fact that no tooth structure is reduced to achieve tooth whitening. A third major advantage of using bleaching to acquire lighter teeth is the fact there is no need for continuous replacement, as with restorative alternatives. Furthermore, there will be no chipping or fracturing of the natural bleached teeth, as tends to occur with restorative modalities (especially bonding, but also with laminating or crowning). Many patients also appreciate the minimal office time made possible by combining an initial in-office procedure (which produces immediately gratifying improvement in lightness) with dentist-monitored home bleaching as described in Chapter 4.

For most dentists, bleaching's chief advantage is its minimal invasiveness, which requires no alteration of tooth structure or loss of enamel yet produces the desired improvement in appearance (Figs 1-8a and 1-8b).

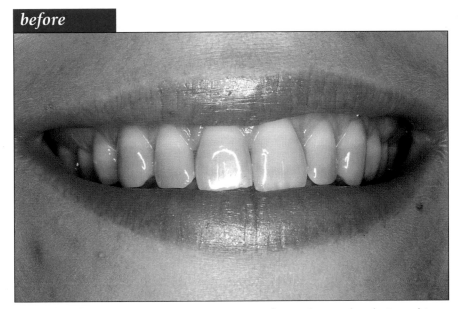

Fig 1-8a The most conservative treatment for patients who desire whiter teeth can begin with bleaching.

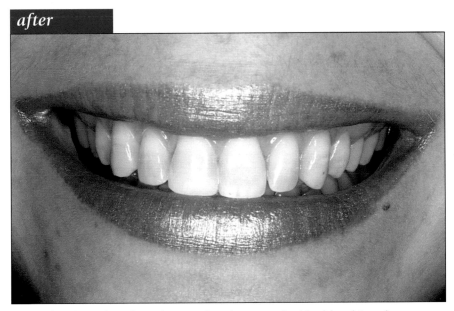

Fig 1-8b Discolored teeth can often be remedied by bleaching alone.

Disadvantages of Bleaching Used Alone

First, the effect of bleaching on natural teeth is not permanent, compared to crowns and veneers, which can be restored to their original brightness through cleaning. This is particularly significant when the staining is caused by behaviors the patient is unwilling to give up, such as smoking or drinking coffee and tea.

Second, it requires more than one or two sessions. Compared to bonding, for instance, the average patient may need to return for several sessions of in-office bleaching.

Third, it is not effective for all forms of discoloration, such as the banding seen in severe tetracycline staining (Fig 1-9a). The banding effect will remain, albeit somewhat lighter in color. However, depending on both lip line and amount of tooth structure revealed during smiling, bleaching can sometimes serve as a compromise treatment (Fig 1-9b). Bleaching also cannot totally correct opacity or white spots frequently seen in fluorosis. While the white areas may be less noticeable on a brightened tooth, they can be hidden completely only by removal or some type of restorative endeavor. Furthermore, bleaching cannot alter the shape or form or position of a tooth, as can be done with bonding, laminating, or crowns.

Fourth, bleaching is inappropriate and even dangerous for some problems. For example, bleaching is contraindicated when the surface, thickness, and health of the enamel has been compromised for any reason, ranging from microcracks that have allowed the stain to permeate the tooth or thinned enamel seen in many systemic diseases or in some older persons.

Fifth, bleaching can be somewhat unpredictable and change "the balance of the smile." If the patient has noticeable amalgams in the area to be bleached, for example, these will have to be removed, since the color difference would be even more apparent after bleaching, necessitating amalgam replacement (see Fig 1-6).

Many of these disadvantages, except for those involving damaged enamel, apply only to bleaching used alone. While they are not necessarily contraindications, they are indicators that bleaching serves best as an adjunct to other esthetic dental treatments. Chapters 3 and 7 explain in detail how this works and where bleaching belongs in the sequence of treatment.

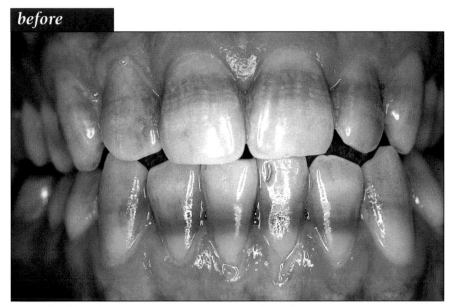

Fig 1-9a This 31-year-old man has severe Class 3 tetracycline staining. Whereas normal bleaching treatments could not achieve the tooth color most people would desire, this patient wanted to try the more conservative treatment first.

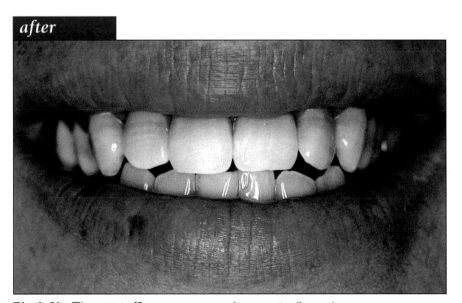

Fig 1-9b Three in-office treatments plus matrix (home) treatments accomplished the result seen here. Because his normal smile line masked most of the problem, the patient was pleased with bleaching therapy alone.

Advantages of Incorporating Bleaching into Combined Therapy

First, adding bleaching to a long-term treatment plan provides immediate improvement in the smile for patients going through other treatments such as orthodontics, periodontics, or implants, and waiting for the final restorative phase incorporating permanent treatments such as porcelain laminates or crowns.

Second, bleaching improves the effect of combined treatment in a variety of ways. For example, lighter shades of crowning or veneering can be used after bleaching other teeth in the arch, then matching this lighter shade. Bleaching all but a single compromised tooth, which can instead be bonded, maximizes effect and minimizes office time and patient expense.

Disadvantages of Incorporating Bleaching into Broader Treatment Plans

These are few. For the patient, adding other treatments generally adds to the office time and cost required. For the dentist, a combination of approaches requires more extensive planning and careful attention to the complexities of matching colors. This is especially important when using bleaching, since the final result is not evident while the patient is in the operatory chair for in-office bleaching and is not completely under the dentist's control when matrix bleaching is used. Chapters 3 and 4 address these problems.

Other obstacles include:

- Increased cost in equipment and office time and training. In spite of increasingly sophisticated heat-light instrumentation, bleaching requires a team approach for maximum effectiveness and safety.

- The lack of complete predictability, which means the effectiveness of bleaching in any specific patient will depend on individual variables. Some of these cannot be determined precisely, such as the cause of the stain and where, how deeply, or how long the stain has permeated the structure of the tooth. The resulting variable degree of improvement is not so significant when bleaching is used alone, but is important when trying to match restorations or other dental treatment, which can be complicated.

- The *relative* impermanence of bleaching. When used in conjunction with more long-lasting treatments, such as bonding, periodic rebleaching of the natural teeth to retain a color match will be an ongoing need.

Creating a Dental Team to Help Shape and Meet Increased Patient Expectations

Bleaching is an appropriate adjunct to cosmetic contouring, orthodontics (especially in the 25% of all orthodontic patients who are adults), periodontal surgery (particularly when used for esthetic reasons such as correcting loss of interdental space or high lip line), orthognathic surgery, and plastic and reconstructive surgery. One of the unexpected advantages of using bleaching with these procedures is that it creates new communication, understanding, and referral patterns between many different specialists.

We are beginning to see the dentist become the initial healthcare provider to whom people bring their wishes, sometimes expressed quite tentatively, for a more attractive appearance. Thanks to innovative materials and technology in dentistry, including increasingly sophisticated computer systems, you can be the person who advises your patient on the multitude of possibilities. You can be the professional who assembles the dental, medical, and sometimes other professionals to achieve the patient's desires. You can appropriately involve and refer to colleagues in related specialties such as periodontics, orthognathic surgery, plastic and reconstructive surgery, and dermatology, as well as other areas concerned with appearance. You will let these specialists know how your esthetic skills can enhance the appearance of their patients seeking specialty care.

References

1. Arens D. The rold of bleaching in esthetics. Dent Clin North Am, 1989;33:319.

2. Mello HS. The mechanism of tetracycline staining in primary and permanent teeth. J Dent Child 1967;34:478.

3. Cohen S, Parkins FM. Bleaching tetracycline-stained vital teeth. Oral Surg 1970;29:465–471.

4. Jordan RE, Boksman L. Conservative vital bleaching treatment of discolored dentition. Compend Contin Ed Dent 1984;5(10):803–808.

5. Chung HY, Bowles WH. Oxidative changes in minocycline leading to intrinsic dental staining. J Dent Res 1989;68 (special issue):413.

6. Dodson DL, Bowles WH. Production of minocycline pigment by tissue extracts. J Dent Res 1991;70:424.

7. Black GV, McKay FS. Mottled teeth: An endemic devlopmental imperfection of the enamel of the teeth heretofore unkown in the oliterature of dentistry. Dent Cosmos 1916;58:129.

8. Murrin JR, Barkmeier WW. Chemical treatment of endemic dental fluorosis. Quintessence Int 1982;13;363–369.

9. Goldstein RE. Bleaching teeth: New materials, new role. J Am Dent Assoc 1987: Dec(special issue):44E–52E.

10. Dzierack J. Factors which cause tooth color changes: Protocol for in-office "power bleaching." Pract Periodont Aesthet Dent 1991;3(2):15–20.

11. Zaragoza VMT. Bleaching of vital teeth: technique. EstoModeo 1984;9:7–30.

12. Zack L, Cohen G. Pulp response to externally applied heat. Oral Surg 1965;19:515–530.

13. Pearson H. Bleaching of the discolored pulpless tooth. J Am Dent Assoc 1958;56:64–68.

14. Nutting EB, Poe GS. A new combination for bleaching teeth. Dent Clin North Am 1976;10:655–662.

15. Baumgartner JC, Reid DE, Pickett A. Human pulpal reaction to the modified McInnes bleaching technique. J Endodont 1983;9:527–529.

16. Bowles WH, Thompson LR. Vital bleaching: The effects of heat and hydrogen peroxide on pulpal enzymes. J Endodont 1986;12(3):108–112.

17. Cohen SC, Chase C. Human pulpal response to bleaching procedures on vital teeth. J Endodont 1979;5;134–138.

18. Griffin RE, Grower, MF. Effects of solutions used to treat dental fluorosis on permeability of teeth. J Endodont 1977;11:391–343.

19. Ledoux W, et al. Structural effects of bleaching on tetracycline stained vital rat teeth. J Prosthet Dent, 1985;54:55–59.

20. Lisanti VF, Zander HA. Thermal injury to normal dog teeth. J Dent Res 1952;31;548–558.

21. Nyborg H, Branstrom M. Pulp reaction to heat. J Prosthet Dent 1968;19:605–612.

22. Postle HH et al. Pulp response to heat. J Dent Res 1959;38:740.

23. Sakaguchi RL, Hampel AT. Bleaching of vital teeth. Clark's Clin Dent 1991, vol 4:1–10.

24. Haywood VB. Bleaching of vital and nonvital teeth. Curr Opin Dent 1992:(March):142–149.

25. Seale NS, McIntosh JE, Taylor AN. Pulpal reaction to bleaching of teeth in dogs. J Dent Res 1981;60:948–953.

26. Garber DA, Goldstein RE, Goldstein CE, Schwartz CG. Dentist-monitored bleaching: A combined approach. Pract Periodont Aesthet Dent 1991;3(2):22–26.

Chemistry of Bleaching

Howard Frysh, BDS, DDS

Bleaching is a chemical process for whitening materials which is widely used in industry. In dentistry, bleaching usually refers to products containing some form of hydrogen peroxide.

The three most prominent commercial bleaching processes are peroxide, chlorine, and chloride, in that order.[1]

Peroxide bleaching requires the least time and is most commonly used. The strength is designated most frequently by volume rather than by percentage of peroxide. Thus, although they are interrelated proportionately, 27.5% hydrogen peroxide is termed 100 volume, 35% is 130 volume, and 50% is 200 volume, volume indicating the volume of oxygen released by one volume of the designated hydrogen peroxide.

Although bleaching processes are complex, the vast majority work by oxidation, the chemical process by which organic materials are eventually converted into carbon dioxide and water. Wood burning in a fireplace is a common example of oxidation. The differences between the oxidation that occurs with bleaching and that of burning wood are the rate of each reaction and the number of intermediate products produced. Burning rapidly transforms a substance into carbon dioxide, water, and heat. In comparison, bleaching slowly transforms an organic substance

25

into chemical intermediates that are lighter in color than the original. Corrosion of metal is an example of a slow oxidation process. If allowed to progress long enough, however, both burning and bleaching will result in the conversion of organic materials into carbon dioxide and water.

The oxidation-reduction reaction which takes place in the bleaching process is known as a *redox reaction*. In a redox reaction the oxidizing agent (eg, hydrogen peroxide) has free radicals with unpaired electrons, which it gives up, becoming reduced; the reducing agent (the substance being bleached) accepts the electrons and becomes oxidized.

Hydrogen Peroxide Bleaching

Hydrogen peroxide is an oxidizing agent and has the ability to produce free radicals, $HO_2\bullet + O\bullet$, which are very reactive ($HO_2\bullet$ is the stronger free radical). In pure aqueous form, hydrogen peroxide is weakly acidic (to reduce breakdown and extend shelf life) and ionizes as shown in Fig 2-1.

The result is that a larger proportion of the weaker free radical $O\bullet$ is produced. The perhydroxyl $HO_2\bullet$ is the more potent free radical. In order to promote the formation of $HO_2\bullet$ ions the H_2O_2 needs to be made alkaline. The optimum pH for this to occur is at a pH of 9.5 to 10.8.

In the ionization of buffered hydrogen peroxide in this pH range (Fig 2-2), a greater amount of perhydroxyl $HO_2\bullet$ free radicals are produced, which results in a greater bleaching effect in the same time as at other pH levels.[2,3] Thus, hydrogen peroxide is most effective between pH 9.5 and pH 10.8.

In the presence of decomposition catalysts and enzymes, the hydrogen peroxide ionization occurs as follows[4]:

$$2H_2O_2 \rightarrow 2H_2O + O_2.$$

This changes the reaction so that no free radicals are produced, rendering the hydrogen peroxide ineffective as a bleaching agent. These enzymes, some of which are present in the mouth, are an important part of the body's defense against oxygen toxicity. It is thus important to have teeth dry and free of debris when applying a bleaching agent.

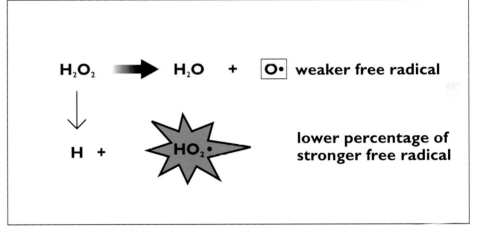

Fig 2-1 Ionization of hydrogen peroxide at acidic pH.

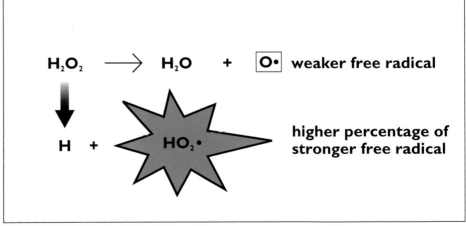

Fig 2-2 Ionization of buffered hydrogen peroxide (pH 9.5 to 10.8).

Dental Bleaching Mechanism

In dental bleaching (Fig 2-3), hydrogen peroxide diffuses through the organic matrix of the enamel and dentin.[5-9] Because the radicals have unpaired electrons, they are extremely electrophilic and unstable and will attack most other organic molecules to achieve stability, generating other radicals. These radicals can react with most unsaturated bonds, resulting in disruption of electron conjugation and a change in the absorption energy of the organic molecules in tooth enamel. Simpler molecules that reflect less light are formed, creating a successful whitening action. This process occurs when the oxidizing agent (hydrogen peroxide) reacts with organic material in the spaces between the inorganic salts in tooth enamel.

A simple example of this type of reaction is the oxidation of beta carotene, which is deep red. When oxidized, this molecule is split in half to produce two molecules of vitamin A, which are colorless (Fig 2-4). However, not all bleaching (oxidizing) reactions are this simple.

A more extensive bleaching process has been described by Albers[10]: "the extent of bleaching . . . determines the amount of whitening compared to the amount of material loss. During the initial bleaching process highly pigmented carbon-ring compounds are opened and converted into chains which are lighter in color. Existing carbon double-bond compounds, usually pigmented yellow, are converted into hydroxy groups (alcohol like), which are usually colorless. As these processes continue the bleached material continually lightens."

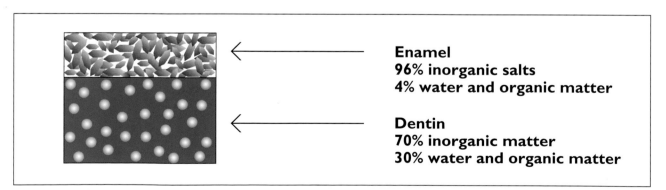

Enamel
96% inorganic salts
4% water and organic matter

Dentin
70% inorganic matter
30% water and organic matter

Fig 2-3 Diffusion of hydrogen peroxide through the organic matrix of enamel and dentin in teeth.

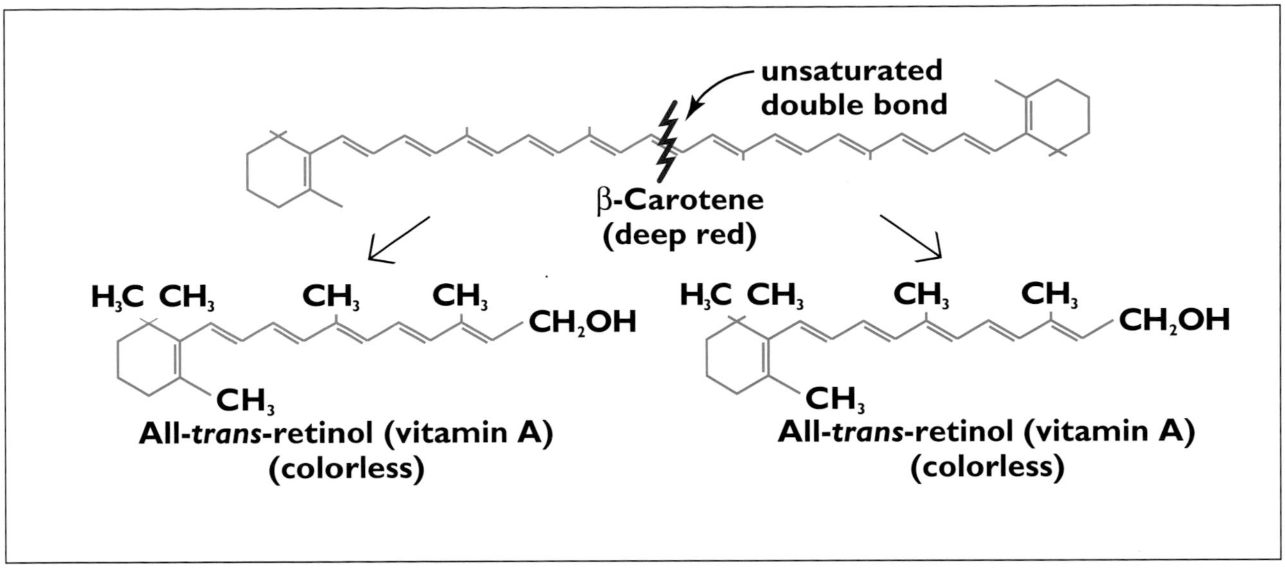

Fig 2-4 Oxidation of beta carotene. A free radical acts at the unsaturated (double) bond (jagged line), producing two molecules of colorless vitamin A.

Saturation Point

As bleaching proceeds, a point is reached at which only hydrophilic colorless structures exist. This is a material's *saturation point.* Lightening then slows down dramatically, and the bleaching process, if allowed to continue, begins to break down the carbon backbones of proteins and other carbon-containing materials. Compounds with hydroxy groups (usually colorless) are split, breaking the material into yet smaller constituents. Loss of enamel becomes rapid, with the remaining material being quickly converted into carbon dioxide and water.[10]

During actual bleaching, all of these reactions occur at the same time, since most materials contain varying amounts of simple and complex chemical components. However, since some processes occur more easily and quickly than others, the rate of each chemical reaction changes as the bleaching process continues. Figure 2-5 illustrates the most common oxidation processes associated with bleaching organic materials. These reactions are common to all proteins, including those of the enamel matrix.[10] The saturation point is located in the middle of the illustration.

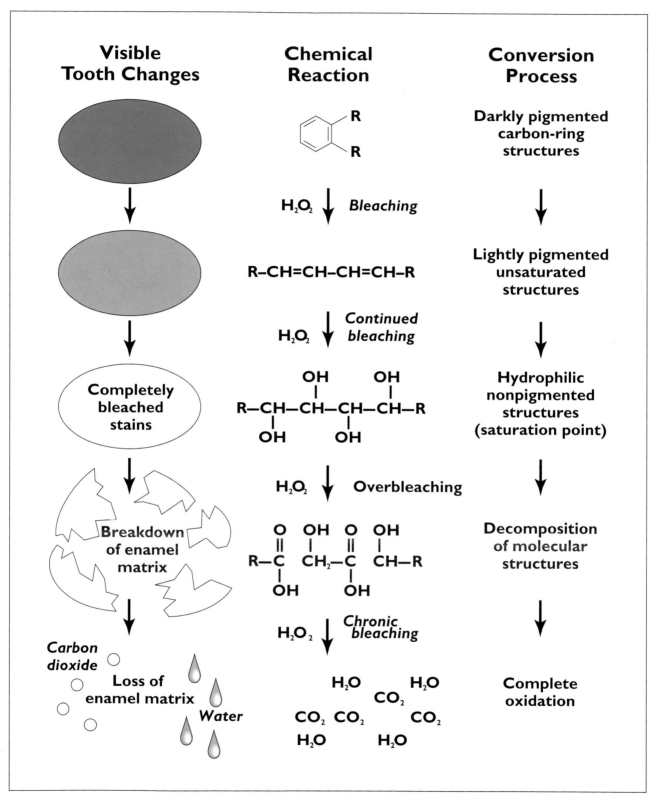

Fig 2-5 Common oxidation processes associated with bleaching teeth. The saturation point, at which the optimal amount of bleaching has occurred, is located in the middle of the diagram. (Reprinted with permission from: Lightening natural teeth. ADEPT Report 1991;2(1):1–24.)

The ultimate result of bleaching processes is, like other oxidation processes, breakdown and loss of tooth enamel. It is therefore critical for the dentist to know that bleaching must be stopped at or before the saturation point, since the price of material loss (tooth brittleness and increased porosity) would then be greater than any marginal gain in tooth whitening. Optimal bleaching achieves maximum whitening, while overbleaching degrades tooth enamel without further whitening.

Carbamide Peroxide Chemistry

Carbamide peroxide is available in concentrations of 3% to 15%. In dental bleaching, carbamide peroxide is usually used at a concentration of 10% to 15%. The carbamide peroxide breaks down into hydrogen peroxide; 10% carbamide peroxide produces 3.6% hydrogen peroxide. Carbamide peroxide breaks down as shown in Fig 2-6. The resulting hydrogen peroxide then ionizes as shown in Figs 2-1 and 2-2.

Carbamide peroxide products contain either a carbopol or glycerine base. The carbopol base slows the release of hydrogen peroxide (Fig 2-7), but this does not change the efficiency of the bleaching treatment.[11] Carbamide peroxide bleaching preparations have a slightly acidic pH to extend shelf life.

As shown in Fig 2-2, the increase in the formation more active perhydroxyl radical ($HO_2 \cdot$) is achieved by buffering the hydrogen peroxide–containing solution.

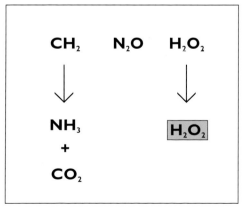

Fig 2-6 Chemical breakdown of carbamide peroxide.

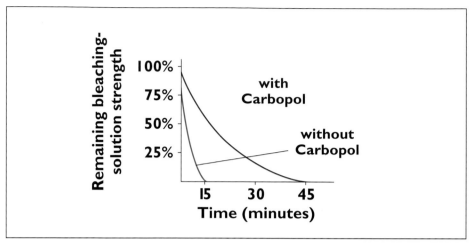

Fig 2-7 Increase in length of bleaching-solution strength for carbamide peroxide bleaching preparations with carbopol vs those without carbopol. (Reprinted with permission from: Lightening natural teeth. ADEPT Report 1991;2(1):1–24.)

Factors That Affect Bleaching

1. *Surface debridement:* Thorough scaling and polishing should be performed in order to eliminate all superficial debris.

2. *Hydrogen peroxide concentration:* The higher the concentration, the greater the effect of the oxidation process. The highest concentration generally used is 35% hydrogen peroxide.[3] *Note*: When gelling agents are added to a 35% solution of hydroden peroxide, the concentration of H_2O_2 is then reduced to 25%.

3. *Temperature:* An increase of 10°C doubles the rate of the chemical reaction. Generally, if the temperature is elevated to a point at which the patient does not feel discomfort, then the procedure is taking place at a safe range of temperature.[12–15]

4. *pH:* When hydrogen peroxide is stored and shipped, an acidic pH must be maintained to extend shelf life. The optimum pH for hydrogen peroxide to have its oxidation effect is pH 9.5 to pH 10.8. This produces a 50% greater result in the same amount of time as at a lower pH.[2,3]

5. *Time:* The effect of the bleach is directly related to the time of exposure. The longer the exposure, the greater the color change.[15]

6. *Sealed environment:* Placing the hydrogen peroxide into a sealed environment has been shown to increase its bleaching efficiency.[1]

References

1. Trotman ER. Dyeing and chemical technology of treatable fibers. In: McGraw-Hill Encyclopedia of Science and Technology, vol 2, ed 6. New York: McGraw Hill, 1987.

2. Frysh H, Bowles W, Baker F, Rivera-Hidalgo G, Guillen G. Effect of pH on bleaching efficiency [abstract 2248]. J Dent Res 1993; 72:384.

3. Zaragoza VMT. Bleaching of vital teeth: Technique. Estomodeo 1984;9:7–30.

4. Carlsson J. Salivary peroxidase: An important part of our defense against oxygen toxicity. J Oral Pathol 1987;16:412–416.

5. Bowles WH, Ugwuneri Z. Pulp chamber penetration by hydrogen peroxide following bital bleaching procedures. J Endodont 1987; 13:375–377.

6. Fuss A, Szajkis S, Tagger M. Tublar permeability to calcium hydroxide and the bleaching agents. J Endodont 1989;15:362–364.

7. Bartelstone HJ. Radioiodine penetration through intact enamel with uptake by bloodstream and thyroid gland. J Dent Res 1951: 30:728–733.

8. Bowles WH, Thompson LR. Vital bleaching: The effect of heat and hydrogen peroxide on pulpal enzymes. J Endodont 1986;12:108–112.

9. Cooper JS, Bokmeyer TJ, Bowles WH. Penetration of the pulp chamber by carbamide peroxide bleaching agents. J Endodont, in press.

10. Albers H. Lightening natural teeth. ADEPT Report 1991;2(1):1–24.

11. Haywood V. Nightguard vital bleaching: Current information and research. Esthet Dent Update 1990;1(2):20–25.

12. Cohen SC. Human pulpal response to bleaching procedures on vital teeth. J Endodont 1979;5:134–138.

13. Robertson WD, Melfi RC. Pulpal response to vital bleaching procedures. J Endodont 1980;6:645–649.

14. Seale NS, McIntosh JE, Taylor AN. Pulpal reaction to bleaching of teeth in dogs. J Dent Res 1981;60:948–953.

15. Fasanara RS. Bleaching teeth: History, chemicals, and methods used for common tooth discolorations. J Esthet Dent 1991;4(3):71–78.

3

Diagnosis and Treatment Planning

Patient Selection

Diagnosis of the etiology of tooth discoloration is the most important determinant of the success of any tooth bleaching. The next most important predictive factor is the condition of the teeth and mouth, especially the presence of compromised teeth that would prohibit the use of either bleaching agents or increased temperatures. But success with bleaching, as measured by immediate and longer-term patient satisfaction, will also depend on many other more personal factors: the individual patient's desires and expectations about the esthetic outcome; willingness to spend time in the dental chair and/or to cooperate at home; and acceptance of responsibility to modify behaviors that can affect tooth coloration.

Determining the Etiology of Discoloration

As previously described, most discoloration falls primarily into one of three categories. The most common staining is *extrinsic*, which tends to be superficial, resulting from excessive use of food substances such as coffee, tea, highly colored food, or tobacco. *Intrinsic* stains are discolorations of the tooth structure that may occur due to ingestion of certain drugs during critical periods of tooth development, excessive exposure to fluorides, or exposure to dental restorative materials. In rare cases, endogenous stains are associated with genetic conditions. The third category, *age-related discoloration,* usually results from a combination of extrinsic staining, thinned enamel, and darkened dentin, all of which occur progressively with age.

Some problems, such as tetracycline staining, are highly variable in extent, coloration, depth of stain, location, and pattern. This variability affects how well a particular problem responds to bleaching. The patient may require a different number of sessions or be better treated through a process of combination bleaching. Many of the rarer causes of discoloration are usually genetic and usually involve altered tooth structure.[1]

Preparation For Bleaching

Visual examination
A thorough visual examination will generally indicate the cause of the dental staining and the extent and depth of discoloration, according to the descriptions outlined in Chapter 1.

Behavioral history
Ask your patient about previous and current use of tobacco, coffee or tea, and highly colored beverages and foods. If you notice microcracks or other structural problems, also ask about habits such as eating ice or chewing on objects like pencils or eyeglasses.

Medical history
Focus on any systemic problems or medications that might have affected or be affecting tooth coloration. Since many such problems begin during critical periods of tooth development, this history needs to be investigated through the prenatal period. Use the following short questionnaire as a guide. Begin by assuring the patient that these questions are asked of all patients to obtain information on possible causes for any discoloration. Explain that questions about where they have lived relate to varying levels of water fluoridation in different areas.

Medical History Questionnaire

1. As far as you know, was your mother ever ill enough to take medicine during her pregnancy with you? If so, which medications?
2. Was there was any Rh incompatibility when you were born? Did you have severe jaundice as an infant? Was there ever a period of nutritional deprivation in your childhood?
3. Have you ever been told you had any of the following medical conditions?
   - any genetic diseases (diseases you were born with)?
   - cerebral palsy? • serious renal damage? • severe allergies?
4. Did you ever have a head or neurological injury in your childhood or adolescence?
5. During your childhood or adolescence, did you ever take antibiotics for cystic fibrosis, Rocky Mountain Spotted Fever, acne, or for any other prolonged period that comes to mind?
6. What parts of the country have you lived in? Do you remember if the level of fluoride was said to be high where you grew up?

Recording of baseline data

We strongly recommend incorporating an intraoral video camera into your practice, both for its expanded diagnostic capabilities and for its value in patient communication[2] described later in this chapter. Commercially available cameras range from self-contained models to those used with computer image-modification systems.[3] The more that a camera is integrated into the evaluation phases of a practice, the greater its benefits will be.[4]

If you are not using an intraoral video camera, photograph any staining at this time, preferably using a high-quality 35-mm camera. These photographs will provide an excellent record of the pretreatment state, which will make it easier to determine proper follow-up. It also will help the patient to later recall how he or she looked before any treatment and to recognize the cumulative effect of what may be a gradual improvement in tooth color.

General oral examination

If the patient has not been under your dental care or or has not been recently evaluated, perform a comprehensive examination of both soft and hard tissues, plus a complete radiographic analysis. McLaughlin and Freedman contend that this is a good time to determine and enhance the patient's "dental IQ" about oral hygiene and dental health, since the patient obviously is acutely conscious of at least one of the benefits of dental health: white teeth.[5]

Determining soundness of individual teeth

The last dental exam should have been recent enough and thorough enough to ascertain the presence of any possible periapical or other pathological condition, caries or defective restorations, and any enlargement of the pulp that may make a tooth unusually sensitive to the planned or contemplated bleaching technique. Recently completed restorations or orthodontics can also result in a hypersensitive pulp which may be more sensitive to bleaching.

The appropriateness of bleaching for vital teeth will depend not only upon the type and severity of stain, but also upon the unbroken surface, thickness, and other measures of the health of the enamel. Discolorations of vital teeth should usually be addressed from the enamel surface, with definitive limits on chemical and heat application. For nonvital teeth, there is less concern for damage to the nonexistent pulp. Tooth integrity is still important, however, as these teeth can be treated from either the inside of the pulp chamber or from the surface, using higher-concentration bleaching agents and more intense heat than for vital teeth.

The presence of microcracks is not necessarily a contraindication to bleaching, but must be carefully considered and measured (Fig 3-1). Deep microcracks may let the bleaching solution enter too deeply into the tooth, causing substantial pain. But even shallower microcracks may affect the results of bleaching by creating a prismatic effect, in which the area around the microcrack is lighter due to the deeper absorption of the bleaching solution. The uneven color thus created can detract from the overall appearance of the tooth.

An intraoral camera can be one of the most important tools in the examination process. Even the most highly trained eye may not see microcracks and other potential deformities as well as a camera. An intraoral camera can be especially effective both for seeing these defects clearly and for documenting them with printouts or video recordings for communication with the patient (Figs 3-2a and 3-2b).

Transillumination techniques also can reveal caries, microcracks, decalcified or hypocalcified areas, and areas of excess calcification, as well as permitting views of the teeth from different angles to observe the opacity, depth, and layers of any stains.

Verifying the vitality of teeth

This is a particularly important step prior to bleaching. If thermal sensitivity was noted at an earlier examination, assess for any changes. If any microcracks were observed, test for sensitivity using ice, cold water, air, and heat, in that order. Radiographs and thermal and electric pulp testing may be necessary to answer questions of pulp vitality that will help determine the type of bleaching procedures to be used. Figure 3-3 illustrates a situation in which a localized stain should first be removed before internal bleaching is performed.

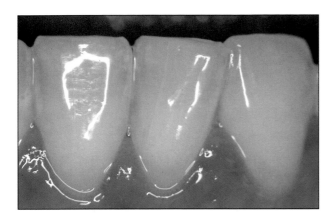

Fig 3-1 Microcracks as seen on these lower incisors are not necessarily a contraindication to bleaching.

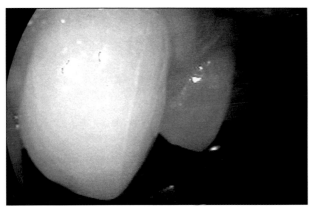

Fig 3-2a This microcrack is visible with the aid of an intraoral video camera.

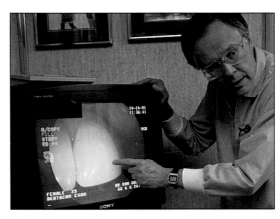

Fig 3-2b The enlarged video picture makes it easy to explain how a microcrack can affect the tooth.

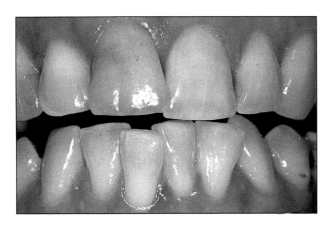

Fig 3-3 This nonvital tooth also has localized staining due to recurrent caries. It should first be treated by replacement of the defect before bleaching. The localized stain should be mechanically removed before the tooth is internally bleached.

Step 8

Complete prophylaxis

A thorough prophylaxis, often including the use of a Prophy-Jet 30 (Dentsply), will enable you to see more clearly the extent of deep stains and to better prepare the teeth for treatment.

When Bleaching May Not Be Necessary

A thorough prophylaxis using the Prophy-Jet at times may remove enough of the extrinsic stain, calculus, and plaque to satisfy some patients without further bleaching.

In other cases, correction of dental restorative problems contributing to discoloration may make bleaching unnecessary. Bacterial degradation of food debris in areas of tooth decay or decomposing fillings can cause deep brown to black discolorations. Other causes are caries and leaking or degraded tooth-colored restorations such as acrylics, glass ionomers, or composites, pictured in Figs 1-5a and 1-5b. All such problems must be corrected before beginning bleaching, which in some cases repair may make superfluous.

If the darkness in teeth is caused by shadowing cast through the enamel by silver, gold, or other metal restorations (see Fig 1-6), replacing these restorations with less visible materials such as composite resin often changes the appearance of the tooth sufficiently to satisfy the patient without bleaching.

When Bleaching May Be Contraindicated

For bleaching of vital teeth, contraindications include:

- Extremely large pulps, which may precipitate sensitivity.
- Other causes of hypersensitivity, such as exposed root surfaces (Fig 3-4) or the transient hyperemia associated with orthodontic tooth movement.
- Severe loss of enamel.
- Extensive restorations. Koa et al[6] suggest that bleaching materials should not come in contact with restorative materials. Their study of bleaching chemicals found roughening on contact with most restorative materials, with the greatest damage done to glass ionomer and the least to porcelain. This may be even more significant in matrix bleaching, in which the teeth have a longer exposure to the chemicals (see Chapter 5).

For bleaching of vital or pulpless teeth, contraindications may include the following:

- Pregnancy and nursing. While no studies have looked at possible risk to pregnant women or nursing infants, most dentists suggest women in these situations wait a few months before undertaking elective treatment with strong chemicals.
- Peroxide allergy. A carefully applied rubber dam can help prevent reactions (Fig 3-5).

For power or home bleaching of vital teeth, as described in Chapter 4, there may be yet other contraindications, including:

- Latex allergy, which means a rubber dam cannot be used in power bleaching.
- Transient hypersensitivity that may occur with prolonged application.
- Hypersensitive reactions or allergic reactions caused by extended exposure to chemicals and appliances, such as burning sensation, sore throat, nausea, irritation, or edema.
- Lack of compliance, either through inability or unwillingness to wear the appliance the necessary time.

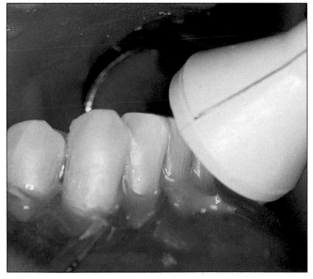

Fig 3-4 For patients with exposed root surfaces that may be hypersensitive, consider using a rubber dam substitute (Den-Mat or Ultradent) to cover these areas. Once the dam is applied, the bleaching can be accomplished normally.

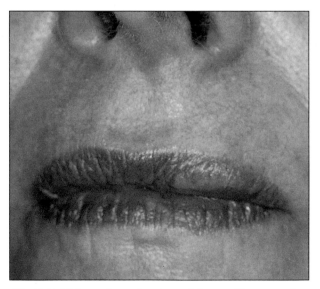

Fig 3-5 This patient developed lip swelling associated with several of the bleaching agents tried during matrix bleaching at home.

When Bleaching Used Alone Is Most Likely to Be an Adequate Treatment

If the patient does not have any of the contraindications listed previously, especially compromised enamel, then the consideration should be whether bleaching used alone will be successful. Generally, the following are good signs:

- Discoloration is fairly light, on the surface, or in the enamel as opposed to the dentin (Figs 3-6a and 3-6b).
- Discoloration on individual teeth is evenly distributed, without dark bands or white spots (Figs 3-7a and 3-7b).
- Teeth are yellowed as their innate color or as a consequence of aging (see Figs 1-7a and 1-7b).
- Discoloration is consistent on all visible teeth, and matching large amalgams or crowns is not required (these can be later replaced to match the lighter colors of successful bleaching).
- Enamel is fairly heavy and even, with no pits, fissures, or grooves.
- There is no need to change tooth structure.

Bleaching used alone, either in-office (Chapter 4) or matrix bleaching (Chapter 5), may also be the treatment of choice for some patients whose teeth do not meet the guidelines given above. While bleaching used alone is less likely to have a maximal effect in such cases, it can still noticeably improve the lightness of the teeth (Figs 3-8a and 3-8b). As the description of patients' "satisfaction quotient" later in this chapter suggests, some patients are willing to forego the better esthetic effect of combined bleaching for the more conservative treatment of bleaching alone. By choosing bleaching alone, they gain the advantages of a shorter time in the dental chair, lower cost, and a very conservative approach with no compromise of tooth structure. This trade-off works only if the

When new restorations are going to be constructed, bleaching should be completed approximately 2 weeks before the final shade selection is chosen for the restoration, since teeth will be unusually bright immediately following bleaching procedures.

patient is fully informed of the limits of the approach and if the patient's acceptance of these limits is fully documented.

When new restorations are going to be constructed, bleaching should be completed approximately 2 weeks before the final shade selection is made for the restoration, since teeth will be unusually bright immediately following bleaching procedures.

Lightening tooth color can be included in a broader treatment plan for improvement of the smile. Because of its simplicity and the relative lack of additional time and expense, bleaching can be a useful part of almost any treatment plan, whether it is periodontal treatment, orthodontics, orthognathic surgery, or plastic and reconstructive surgery (Figs 3-9a and 3-9b). Chapter 7 describes the sequence of treatment in these combinations.

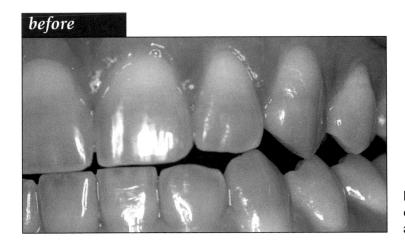

Fig 3-6a Bleaching usually produces more effective, longer lasting results in teeth that are stained slightly yellow or brown.

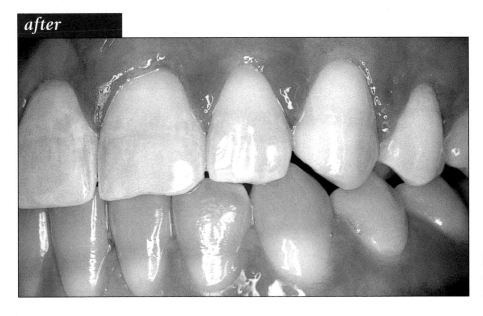

Fig 3-6b After four in-office bleaching treatments, a successful result is obtained.

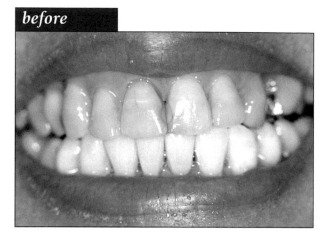

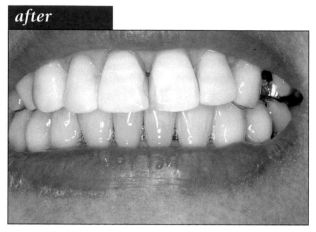

Fig 3-7a Bleaching can be most effective when the discoloration is evenly distributed without dark bands or white spots. The lower teeth have already had one session of in-office bleaching. Note the difference in the discoloration between the two arches.

Fig 3-7b This patient received two in-office bleaching treatments to obtain this result. It is best to wait 2 to 3 weeks before replacing the discolored class 3 restorations.

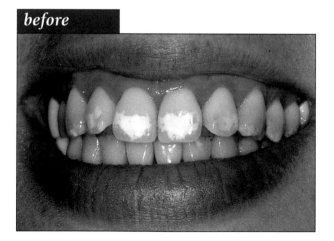

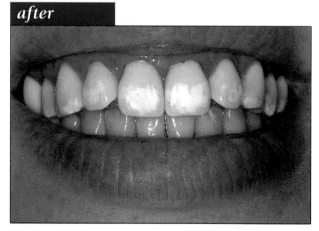

Fig 3-8a The hypocalcified spots on this patient's teeth show up dramatically against the yellow-stained teeth.

Fig 3-8b After three in-office bleaching treatments, note that even though the hypocalcified spots are still present, they are less noticeable. Bonding, laminating, or microabrasion could eliminate them completely if the patient so desires.

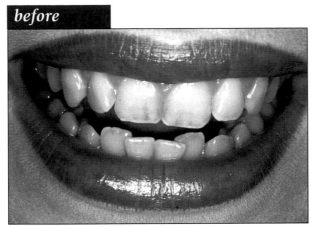

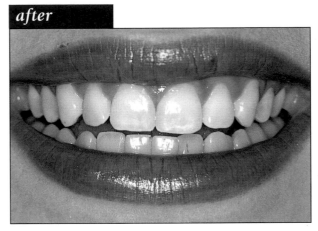

Fig 3-9a This 20-year-old beauty contestant wanted to have the color of her tetracycline-stained teeth improved especially for the statewide Miss America pageant.

Fig 3-9b A combination of in-office bleaching plus minor orthodontics and cosmetic contouring improved her smile in time for the pageant.

Special Considerations for Bleaching in Older Patients

Unless the enamel is very severely worn, bleaching can be an especially effective and appealing treatment for age-related discolorations. Teeth yellowed due to age usually produce the most dramatic bleaching results (see Figs 1-7a and 1-7b). Many older patients appreciate bleaching's shorter chair time, lack of invasiveness, and relatively low cost. The shrinking of the pulp often seen in older patients can make bleaching an especially effective treatment because it is possible to use higher bleaching temperatures than in younger patients.

The type and degree of discolorations in the older patient depend on a mixture of genetics, tooth use and abuse, and habits. Years of smoking and coffee drinking have a cumulative staining effect (see Fig 1-1a), and these and other stains become even more visible because of the inevitable changes on tooth surface, within its crystalline structure, and in the underlying dentin and pulp. In addition to tooth wear and trauma, older amalgams and other restorations begin to degrade.

A thinning of the enamel may cause the facial surface of the tooth to appear flat, with a progressive shift in color due to a loss of the optical reflective properties of the enamel layer. At the same time the enamel begins to thin, secondary dentin formation progresses through a natural protective mechanism in the dentin and pulp. This dentin also begins to darken. The combination of thinned enamel and darkened dentin results in an older-looking tooth. Bleaching can do much to counteract these effects. (If these types of problems occur in a young person, laminating produces a better long-term result.)

Special Considerations for Bleaching in Younger Patients

Children are especially sensitive to any physical characteristic that makes them different or attracts negative attention. This would appear to make children with discolored teeth excellent candidates for bleaching, which does not involve altering a growing tooth. But children may be more difficult candidates for bleaching for the very reason older adults are often good candidates. In children's teeth, the pulps are larger, with little recession or secondary dentin, so they tend to be more sensitive to the thermal stimulation in power bleaching. Bleaching can be done at any age, but greater care must be taken with younger patients in order to avoid pulpal hyperemia. One approach is to minimize or avoid the use of heat, using more lower-intensity in-office sessions or matrix bleaching requiring no heat at all (Fig 3-10).

Even with matrix bleaching, however, children require special attention. Many are less likely to be as attentive to home care as adults. It is imperative that teeth be clean before inserting the matrix; a child with less-than-perfect home care may leave plaque on the teeth and thus diminish the effect of bleaching. These young patients must be made to realize that no bleaching will take effect on a dirty tooth area. A Rotadent or similar plaque-removal device should be used with children using matrix bleaching to require them to clean each individual tooth. Disclosing tablets or solutions also can be an effective tool in helping children see where they are not cleaning properly.

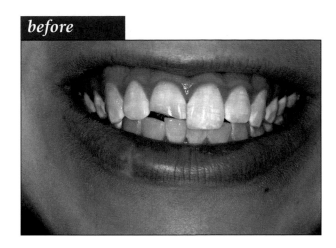
before

Fig 3-10 This 14-year-old boy was embarrassed about the appearance of a fractured tooth, as well as the discoloration of his teeth. Treatment consisted of two in-office treatments without heat, followed by composite resin bonding of the right central incisor. Note the improvement in color between the two arches.

Patient "Warranties": Dealing with Patient Expectations

Patient expectations have changed dramatically in recent years. They expect to live longer and healthier. And they expect to look good doing it.

But, as our colleagues in medicine know all too well, people also often expect health professionals to be able to quickly "fix" problems that may have taken years to develop or for which there is only a partial solution. The dentist interested in esthetics will find a sympathetic ear in the plastic surgeon to whom patients bring photographs of film and television stars and ask for "her nose" or "his chin." It is sometimes hard to explain to a patient why that particular "look" is not right for his or her face. It's even harder to help some patients visualize what you are describing for them. But if you do not succeed, the problems you will face can range from a quietly disappointed patient to a lawsuit. Communication is an essential component of all esthetic endeavors and is greatly facilitated by the visualization offered by computer imaging.

Every patient wants, and in fact is entitled to, some kind of warranty or guarantee of outcome. Bleaching is an inexact science, its result dependent on numerous factors such as the dentist's skill, individual variation in the teeth, and the patient's continuing habits, diet, and hygiene care. It is difficult to guarantee or promise your patient a specific shade or result.

However, every patient wants and expects some forecast by you. If you fail to give the patient a careful, logical contract of what you expect the results of treatment to be, you have by default implied that the results of treatment will be what the patient envisions and that the result will last as long as the patient believes.

The key to avoiding many of the problems of disappointed patients is ensuring that the patient understands all aspects of the problem, the treatment options available, their relative advantages and disadvantages, and just what is involved in keeping the enhanced look for as long as possible.

This provides the patient information necessary to make an informed decision about which, if any, treatment he or she wants. Providing adequate information—and documenting that it has been provided and understood—also protects the dentist. Documentation is essential, because patients, like all of us, sometimes have selective hearing and remember only what they would like the situation to be. In a broad study of patient understanding of esthetic restorative life expectations, Goldstein and Lancaster[7] reported that dentists who explained composite-resin bonding's limited lifetime believed their patients understood this fact. However, a third of the patients convincingly reported that their bonding would last forever, illustrating that patients may remember only what they choose to, or legitimately forget oral estimates of restorative life expectancy.

> *The key to avoiding many of the problems of disappointed patients is ensuring that the patient understands all aspects of the problem, the treatment options available, their relative advantages and disadvantages, and just what is involved in keeping the enhanced look for as long as possible.*

There are three ways to achieve an accurate and documented contract:

1. Collect and document as much information as possible on the patient's smile, the patient's expectations, and what the patient has been told about the possibilities and limitations of various procedures. This documentation process can be done with extensive notetaking and high-quality photographs, but technological advances in imaging and documentation make the process easier and much more accurate.

The most basic of these advanced tools is the extraoral video camera,[2] which can be suspended from a ceiling-mounted, motorized track, mounted above the chair and over the patient's shoulder. When not in use, it can be retracted (Fig 3-11a). As an alternative, a portable video camera, preferably mounted on a tripod, can be used. Videotaping the diagnostic interview provides a complete record of the patient's expectations and preferences and of the dentist's suggestions and explanations of various treatment options, capabilities, and limitations. It also documents the patient's appearance before treatment. In addition to views of the patient's mouth with and without retraction, images should be captured of the patient in right and left oblique views and a center close-up while he or she goes through the motions of speaking and smiling. The anatomic characteristics of the face in motion are far more detailed and useful than still photographs, and will include documentation of details such as the shape of the face, hair and makeup, and any wrinkling or scars.

> *Collect and document as much information as possible on the patient's smile, the patient's expectations, and what the patient has been told about the possibilities and limitations of various procedures.*

The high-quality intraoral video cameras now available enable more precise diagnosis of microcracks and other problems. Often connected to a computer system, these cameras can also be used throughout treatment for visual records of procedural milestones such as preparation and cementation, as well as of any problems encountered. Although an intraoral camera can be used for full-face patient interviews, a ceiling-mounted extraoral camera is less noticeable and intrusive.

2. Share this information with the patient in a way that he or she can visualize its impact on the smile (Fig 3-11b). Our own practice is organized around patient and staff education.[8] We use video-image modification to demonstrate treatment possibilities. We start with a patient's smiling face and electronically experiment with changes such as veneering to mask stains, bonding to close a diastema, correcting the proportions of the smile line, or bleaching. Advances in computer imaging technology have made

a great difference in helping patients visualize, evaluate, and agree to treatment options. Seeing exactly how a smile might be made more esthetically pleasing can also be a powerful marketing aid, overcoming some patients' initial reluctance to invest time and money in a "cosmetic" procedure (Figs 3-11c and 3-11d).

You must be careful, however, not to let a tool designed to improve patient-practitioner communication turn into the cause of later legal disagreements. Most patients are familiar with video-image modification, and some—but certainly not all—may understand from experience (such as at the makeup counter) that the images created are objectives, not precise representations of what can be accomplished. It is important they are told of any limiting factors, such as the location of tooth roots, interarch distance, or possible problems with phonetics and function impairment. Fortunately, many of the new imaging units permit printing a disclaimer statement on the printed image (Fig 3-11e). A videotape of the diagnostic and treatment planning session with the patient will also serve this purpose.

3. Obtain a written "informed patient consent" documenting the patient's understanding and agreement that bleaching may not have precise outcomes. This document could be as simple as a letter to the patient before treatment begins, in which the desired outcome is specified and the potential immediate and long-term limitations are itemized in detail. It could also resemble the more complex informed-consent form patients and practitioners sign before surgery or similar medical procedures. This document would include all possible outcome and treatment problems, such as the unlikely possibility of discomfort, leakage, and allergic reactions.

Such written consent is especially important if the patient is asking for a procedure that the dentist believes has a lesser chance of success or is likely to produce a less-than-desirable result. Patients with this situation are described later in this chapter; also see Figs 7-3a and 7-3b for a good illustration of this kind of case.

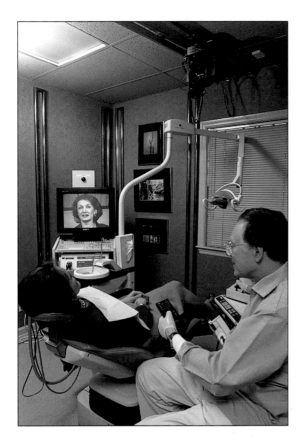

Fig 3-11a A ceiling-mounted remote controlled extraoral video camera (Panasonic D5100) on a motorized track (Telemetrics) can be extremely helpful to record the diagnostic interview. It provides a complete record of the patient's expectations and preferences and of the dentist's explanations of the treatment options, including advantages and limitations of each.

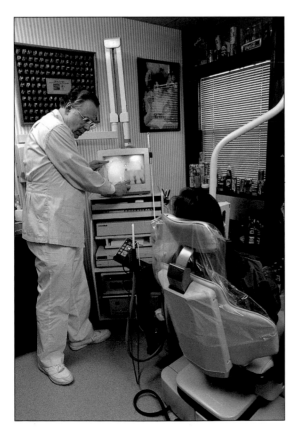

Fig 3-11b Using an intraoral video camera that can record both an enlargement of a patient's tooth and a radiograph (Prodentec, Mobius) can display important diagnostic information to share with the patient.

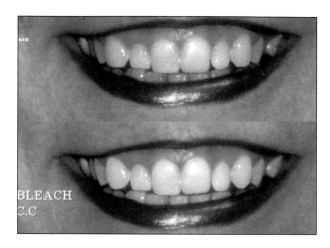

Fig 3-11c This patient was shown her esthetic treatment options using computer imaging. The choice seen here incorporates only bleaching and cosmetic contouring.

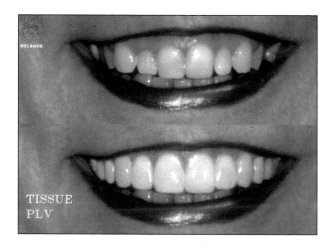

Fig 3-11d The alternative or ideal treatment shown to the patient consisted of maxillary tissue raising and porcelain laminate veneers combined with mandibular bleaching and cosmetic contouring.

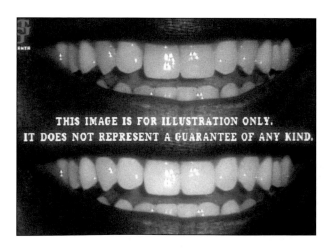

Fig 3-11e Computer imaging is a helpful aid for patients to be able to see relative color differences through tooth bleaching. It is essential to use a disclaimer like the one shown here.

The following questions should provide the basis of your discussions with the patient and your answers should be documented.

1. What will the esthetic result be?

Frequently patients want "white teeth," which to them often means "pure white." This might not be obtainable in their particular situation using bleaching, and, in some cases, might be highly undesirable in relation to skin tone. It is important to show patients the range of lightening expected to occur and to fully explain the limitations of bleaching.

Computer imaging is an excellent means of communicating potential results and of comparing treatment options. Definitive diagnoses are elusive in esthetic dentistry, in large part because each practitioner has his or her own concept of esthetics, which may be quite different from the patient's subjective desire. By placing an image of the patient's face in a computer imaging system, you can demonstrate your concept of the treatment possibilities, and the patient can make alterations to it. Patients may not always know just what they want, but they certainly know what they do not want. It may be necessary to incorporate both practitioner and patient ideas into a composite to satisfy all esthetic and functional needs.[9] Our experience suggests that this is particularly important in esthetic dentistry; patients tend to accept costly treatment options more often when they are satisfied that you understand what they want or expect as a final result.[9]

> *Patients may not always know just what they want, but they certainly know what they do not want.*

2. What will be the costs of the various options?

The patient needs to understand that costs will vary if more bleaching sessions are necessary than anticipated. It is prudent to make any potential extras known to the patient in advance—no surprises!

3. How much office time is involved, both number of visits and hours in the chair per session? For matrix bleaching, how many hours of use per day over how many weeks?

A basic answer is that in-office bleaching usually requires from one to three 90-minute sessions, with darker teeth requiring more sessions. Matrix bleaching usually requires wearing the matrix for 90 minutes daily for 3 to 5 weeks.

4. How soon will results begin to be apparent?

This may be the most important question to answer. Be sure to explain to patients that adequate bleaching often means "overbleaching," since a slight color reversal can be expected within the first few weeks.

5. What is the life expectancy of the change?

It is important that the patient understand that bleaching is not a permanent treatment and that some periodic rebleaching will be required, even if the patient is scrupulously careful to avoid staining agents. Some of the previously oxidized substances may become chemically reduced and cause the tooth to reflect the old discoloration, or the enamel may become remineralized with the staining molecule of the original systemic stain. The patient's acceptance that there will need to be follow-up and retreatment is particularly important with combined bleaching and restorative treatments, since bleaching may lose its effect earlier than adjacent cosmetic restorations. Patients need to know how often retreatment will be required, and what the time and costs are. Usually retreatment can be accomplished with either one in-office session or a 3-week sequence of wearing a matrix once a year. Make certain the patient understands that any retreatment will incur a separate charge, usually at the same cost as the previous bleaching.

6. What behavior patterns must the patient change in order to maintain the improvement?

Patients having matrix bleaching must, of course, comply with the regimen. But patients with any esthetic treatment must fully understand the limitations of the new smile. Continued application of the staining agent in coffee or colored foods, the use of alcohol (which can dissolve bonding agents, veneers, and composites), or the damage done by chewing on objects such as eyeglasses while lost in thought all contribute to degradation of the esthetic treatment.

The Patient's "Satisfaction Quotient"

One of the advantages of going through patient education and complete documentation of a treatment plan is the communication developed between practitioner and patient and the possibility of satisfying the patient's subjective esthetic needs with optimal time and expense. For example, the best treatment for a given patient may be laminates, but the patient may resist, asking instead to try bleaching because of the difference in cost. In this case, we determine a crude "satisfaction quotient" simply by asking the patient if he or she would be satisfied with a certain percentage improvement. Our general rule of thumb is that if the patient believes a 50% improvement would be satisfactory as a trade-off for the less-expensive treatment and if bleaching is not contraindicated and has the potential for "reasonable" esthetic improvement, we document the agreement and proceed. If, on the other hand, the patient determines that he or she would not be satisfied with an improvement at this level, we would suggest electing a more extensive procedure or waiting rather than being disappointed (Figs 3-12a and 3-12b).

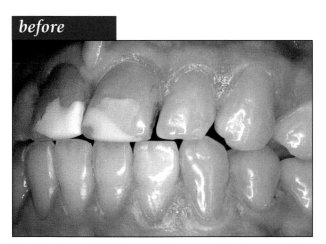

Fig 3-12a This 18-year-old woman had tetracycline stain, as well as hypocalcified white spots on her maxillary central incisors.

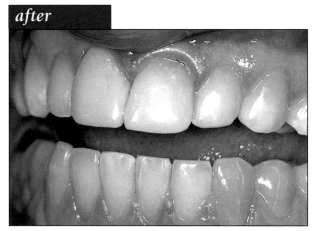

Fig 3-12b The treatment plan consisted of bleaching the teeth in combination with direct bonding of the central incisors. Several in-office bleaching treatments were repeated over the last 14 years to keep the teeth light. Although the patient has been given an option for porcelain laminates, she remains satisfied with the lightness achieved.

The Perfectionist Patient

A patient who is a perfectionist is usually an unlikely candidate for bleaching. Bleaching is an inexact science and results can be unpredictable. But with extensive communication, especially using computer imaging, and with the expanded options of bleaching as a combined therapy, even the perfectionist patient can be satisfied.

References

1. Ishikawa G, Waldron C. Color Atlas of Oral Pathology. St Louis: Ishiyaku EuroAmerica, 1987.

2. Goldstein RE, Miller MC. High technology in esthetic dentistry. Curr Opin Cosmet Dent 1993:5–11.

3. Reis DJ. High-tech trends in dentistry. Dent Prod Rep 1993;27 (5):58–66.

4. Ball MJ, Douglas JV. Informatics in professional education. Meth Informatics Med 1989;28:250–254.

5. McLaughlin G, Freedman G. Color Atlas of Tooth Whitening. St Louis: Ishiyaku EuroAmerica, 1991.

6. Koa EC, Peng P, Johnston WM. Color changes of teeth and restorative materials exposed to bleaching. J Dent Res 1991;70:750.

7. Goldstein RE, Lancaster J. Survey of patient attitudes toward current esthetic procedures. J Prosthet Dent 1984;52:775–780.

8. Goldstein, RE. Change Your Smile, ed 3. Chicago: Quintessence, in press.

9. Goldstein CE, Goldstein RE, Garber DA. Computer imaging: An aid to treatment planning. J Calif Dent Assoc 1991;19(3)47–51.

In-Office Bleaching of Vital Teeth

4

Successful bleaching depends on careful diagnosis and patient selection, as previously described, and on extensive treatment planning to determine how and when bleaching can best be used to maximize the desired esthetic effect and dental health. Some patients will want all their treatment done in the office so they will not be bothered at home. Although it is best to do one arch at a time to keep a control, some patients have such a demanding schedule that it is necessary to bleach both arches simultaneously (Figs 4-1a to 4-1c). Others would prefer to accomplish bleaching entirely by using the matrix technique. However, the most effective result by far will be obtained using a combination of in-office and home procedures.

There are several in-office techniques for bleaching vital teeth, all based on the use of concentrated hydrogen peroxide solution. There are a number of concentrated bleaching gels that can be used; some utilize heat and light to catalyze or speed up the reaction, while others do not. In one instance, the manufacturer suggests a composite curing light for accelerating the bleaching process (Shofu). Although all of the techniques work to varying degrees, there can be a dramatic difference in the bleaching efficiency among them.

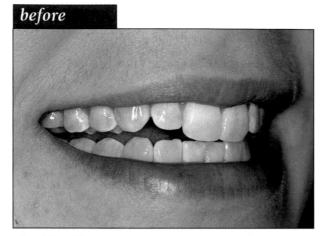

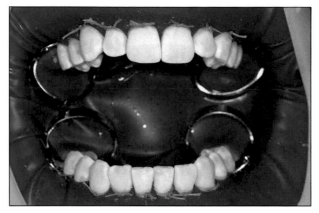

Fig 4-1a This patient was concerned with the yellow stains on her upper and lower teeth.

Fig 4-1b Because of her extremely busy schedule, both arches were bleached during the same in-office appointment.

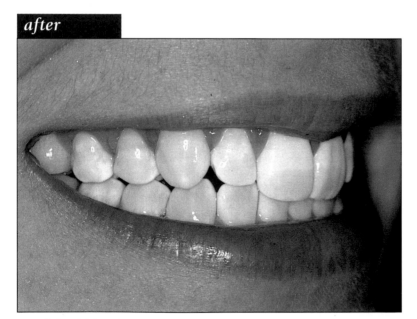

Fig 4-1c Although the teeth were not a perfect color, considerable improvement can be observed above from the in-office treatment.

Bleaching Materials
Bleaching solution. The oldest and standard bleaching agent is a 30% to 35% hydrogen peroxide solution, available in 10-mL prepackaged dosages. These are the most practical for obtaining maximum efficiency and guarding against deterioration of the solution once it is exposed to air.
Bleaching light. Some dentists use a photoflood lamp focused on the labial surface of the teeth, providing light as well as heat. Others prefer a rheostat-controlled solid-state heating device with specially shaped metal tips that provides precise localized heating of the bleaching solution on the teeth. The Illuminator (Union Broach) is a state-of-the-art bleaching instrument combining an activation light source and a metal wand for individual bleaching procedures on both vital and nonvital teeth. A built-in sensor allows for accurate temperature control of the bleaching-light temperature, elevating or lowering it as needed to maintain predetermined thermal levels. Darker teeth or darker sections of teeth can be blended with extra heat by the bleaching wand following a generalized in-office bleaching procedure using the light source.
35-mm camera. A high-quality camera should be used to record progress.
Safety glasses. These should be provided for both for the patient and the entire dental team.

No matter which bleaching procedure is selected, careful preparation and finishing will be needed. The following guidelines cover the basic procedures for bleaching with heat/light or the newer materials that suggest no extra heat to accelerate the bleaching process. The guidelines also have been modified as needed for teeth that are evenly or unevenly stained.

Preparation

The initial pretreatment photographs are taken to be used as baseline data (Fig 4-2a). The teeth must be cleaned of all surface stains and plaque with a Prophy-Jet 30 (Dentsply) or a similar extra cleaning device, as normal prophylaxis pastes are usually not sufficient to remove deeply ingrained stains. This is especially important if your patient has recently completed orthodontic treatment, since band adhesives and cements are difficult to remove and often restain teeth. If there are remnants of bonding material, polish the teeth with an ET 6 or 9 UF 30 blade carbide (Brasseler) until the teeth are free of composite resin.

Step 2

Isolate and protect the teeth and mouth. Apply Oraseal (Ultradent) to gingiva labially, buccally, lingually, and interproximally to protect the soft tissue (Fig 4-2b). The teeth to be bleached should be isolated with a rubber dam and all teeth ligated with waxed dental floss. *Unwaxed dental floss acts as a wick and would absorb the hydrogen peroxide and possibly burn the tissues.* Form a protective pocket by folding back the corners of the rubber dam and apply Oraseal to the linguoproximal surfaces only at the gingival areas to act as an additional seal against leakage. Apply Oraseal to any amalgams present to seal and help block out some of the heat generated by the bleaching light. Using nonmetallic clamps or rubber stops to secure the rubber dam will reduce any possible sensitivity caused by heat buildup in metal clamps (Figs 4-2c and 4-2d).

Step 3

Prepare the teeth by first removing any excess Oraseal from the enamel surface and pumice each tooth to remove any residual sealant or stain (Fig 4-2e). Rinse thoroughly for 10 seconds.

Step 4

For severely stained teeth, etching each tooth facially and lingually for 5 to 7 seconds using 35% phosphoric acid may enhance the penetrability of the bleaching solution and should produce the greatest amount of immediate stain reduction (Fig 4-2f). Rinse and dry the teeth thoroughly (Figs 4-2g and 4-2h). Observe the enamel to make certain that no resin covers any area you intend to bleach.

Step 5

Protect the patient and the dental team from the heat and light involved in bleaching. Explain and emphasize to the patient that he or she must wear safety glasses until you say they can be removed due to the intense light and that his or her hands and clothes must remain under the heavy plastic wrap you will use for a drape since the bleach can burn them. Protect the patient's upper lip and adjacent tissue by placing a piece of gauze saturated with cold water under the rubber dam. Also place gauze saturated with cold water over any metal clamps and the lower lip on top of the dam when bleaching maxillary teeth. Keep these gauze squares wet throughout the bleaching procedure, in order to protect the lips from the increased temperatures generated by the bleaching light.

Do not use any local anesthesia during bleaching. You need the patient's feedback if there is leakage on tissue or if the heat becomes too intense. (Matrix bleaching may be more appropriate for the rare patient who insists on anesthesia.)

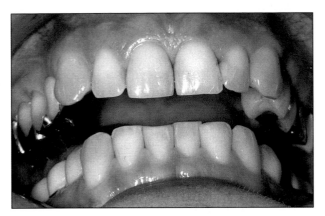
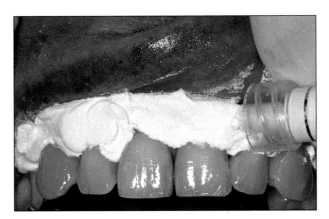

Figs 4-2a and 4-2b This 48-year-old woman wanted a brighter smile and requested an in-office power bleach for rapid results. In order to protect the tissue during bleaching, Oraseal (Ultradent) is generously applied to the gingival areas, both labial and lingual, prior to placement of the rubber dam.

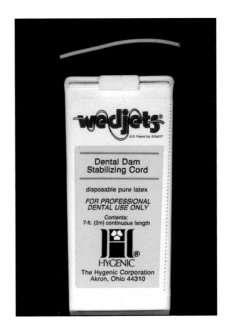
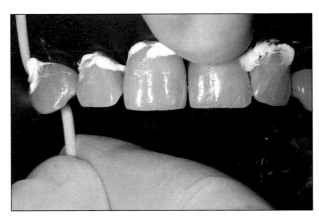

Figs 4-2c and 4-2d A rubber dam clamp is avoided by using elastic rubber stops (Wedjets, Hygenic Corp).

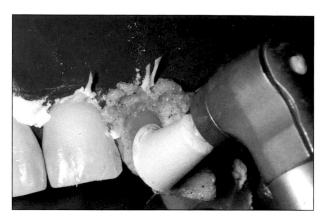

Fig 4-2e Polishing the teeth with coarse pumice removes any extrinsic stains and surplus Oraseal.

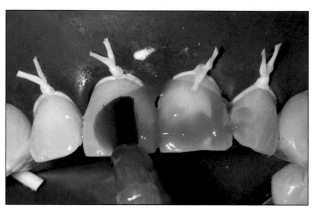

Fig 4-2f In severely stained teeth, etching each tooth facially and lingually for 5 to 7 seconds using 35% phosphoric acid may enhance the penetration of the bleaching solution.

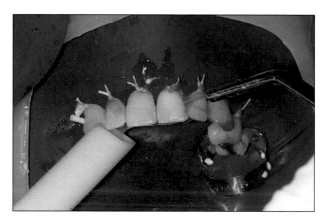

Fig 4-2g The etch solution is immediately washed off using a water syringe and high-volume suction.

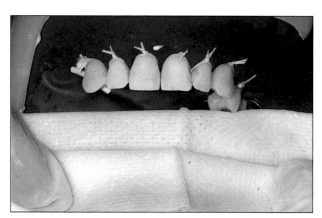

Fig 4-2h Just before bleaching, a folded 2" × 2" gauze pad is placed over the lower lip to contain any extra solution that may drip down.

Application of Bleaching Materials

There are several differences in the actual bleaching procedure depending on the etiology and severity of the discoloration.

1. The number of treatments required will differ. For teeth stained by coffee, tea, or other substances; for many cases of fluorosis-stained teeth; or for the yellowing associated with aging, a dramatic difference can appear in only one or two visits. For tetracycline-stained teeth, three or more visits are generally required, even if combined with an out-of-office matrix technique.

2. The bleaching solution itself will vary, depending on the severity of the stain. For most bleaching, a 30% to 35% concentration of hydrogen peroxide is used, following mild etching to enhance penetrability.

3. The method of applying the bleaching solution to the teeth also will differ, depending on the cause of the discoloration. For evenly distributed extrinsic or tetracycline stains, the bleaching solution is usually applied by infusing gauze draped over the teeth. For the more heterogeneous stains of fluorosis, paint the bleach on the tooth directly in order to localize it according to the pattern of staining.

In most clinical cases, all involved teeth should not be bleached simultaneously. In order to determine the effect of the treatment, some teeth should be left untreated to serve as controls so you can verify the efficacy of the bleaching procedure. Treatment should begin on the most discolored teeth and proceed to the less discolored, using the minimally discolored teeth as a control. Yellow or yellow-brown stains are easier to remove than gray, and the incisal portions of teeth are bleached more quickly than cervical portions, due to thinner dentin and increased thickness of enamel. For fluorosis-stained teeth, there may be unaffected teeth that can be used as controls. For tetracycline-stained teeth and other problems, the mandibular teeth can be used as a control while bleaching the maxillary teeth.

Bleaching with Heat/Light

Homogeneous Discoloration

The application of the bleaching solution is identical for extrinsic staining, tetracycline, minocycline, or other systemic causes of a consistent, homogeneous discoloration.

After rinsing and drying the teeth at the end of the five preparatory steps above, place on the dried teeth a layer of single-thickness cotton gauze that has been saturated with 35% hydrogen peroxide bleaching solution such as Superoxol (Fig 4-2i). The cotton should be cut long and wide enough to cover all of the teeth to be bleached (Fig 4-2j).

Position a bleaching light approximately 13 inches (30 cm) from the teeth to be bleached, and direct the beam directly onto the labial surface of the teeth (Fig 4-2k). Begin with 115°F (consult the light's instruction manual for the proper rheostat setting) and increase the temperature incrementally as long as the patient feels no sensitivity. The bleaching temperature recommended for vital teeth ranges from 115° to 140°F. Temperatures slightly less than 115°F will also catalyze the reaction, but at a slower rate (Fig 4-2l).

Safety note: Care must be taken to prevent irreversible pulp damage from thermal stimulation. The patient's comfort can be used as a guide for increasing or decreasing the temperature administered. A general rule of thumb is to adjust the temperature at least 10 degrees below the temperature at which the patient experiences discomfort (although knowledge of the patient is important, since some patients will suffer silently in their desire to have bright teeth).

Keep the gauze over the teeth being bleached continually saturated and wet with the bleaching agent by dispensing fresh bleaching solution from an eyedropper or cotton swab, and maintain contact of teeth to be bleached with a bleaching agent and heat/light for 20 to 30 minutes.

Remove the gauze and flush the teeth with copious amounts of warm water before carefully removing the floss and rubber dam (Fig 4-2m).

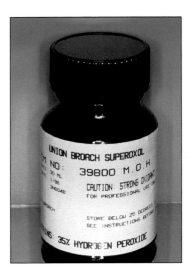

Fig 4-2i Although there are a number of products that can be used as concentrated bleaching agents, this simple 35% hydrogen peroxide solution is often an appropriate choice. (Superoxol, Union Broach)

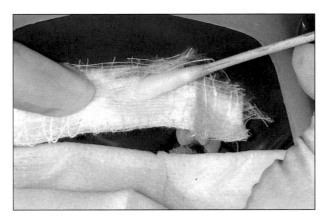

Fig 4-2j A single thickness 2" × 2" gauze pad is saturated with hydrogen peroxide and applied directly on the teeth. A cotton swab is used to continually apply fresh solution.

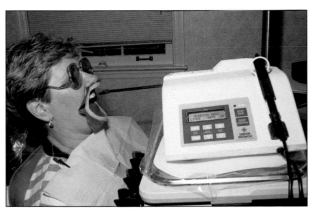

Fig 4-2k The Illuminator (Union Broach) is ideal to use due to its accuracy in recording the bleaching times and temperatures. In addition to a light, it also has an individual wand for extra heat on darkly stained teeth.

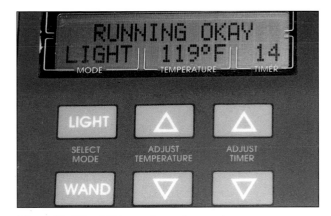

Fig 4-2l The LED readout shows the temperature and time remaining.

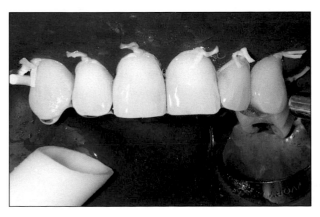

Fig 4-2m After 20 to 30 minutes under the light, the teeth are rinsed with room-temperature water and the dam is removed.

Uneven Discoloration

When extra bleaching is necessary, the application of bleaching solution is similar for fluorosis-stained teeth and other conditions in which only selected teeth are affected or in which the discoloration is uneven on the teeth. The main difference is the extra effort in dealing with the more concentrated stained areas.

 After rinsing and drying at the end of the five preparatory steps listed above, apply a fresh solution of 35% hydrogen peroxide to the stained area of enamel of the teeth exposed through the rubber dam with a cotton-tipped applicator. Allow the solution to remain on the teeth for 5 to 10 minutes.

 Reapply the mixture and immediately disk the enamel with a fine cuttle disk or composite polishing disk.

 Leave this mixture on the enamel, and bleach for 5 minutes with a bleaching light set 13 inches (30 cm) from the teeth to be bleached. Set the rheostat to 115°F and work up to a temperature at which the patient is comfortable, with a maximum of 160°F (see safety note on page 64 concerning heat).

 Repeat the sequence of application of bleach, disking with abrasive disks, and heating with light until the desired shade is obtained. Neutralize the bleaching solution by swabbing with 5.25% sodium hypochlorite and flushing with copious amounts of room-temperature water before removing the rubber dam and any excess Oraseal.

Bleaching Without Heat

Two products contain dual-activated bleaching systems, which lighten the teeth through chemical and light oxidation instead of heat. Hi Lite (Shofu) uses 35% hydrogen peroxide and, typically, a curing light to activate the process. The hydrogen peroxide comes in a powder and liquid that are combined to produce a gel. The gel should be applied in a 1- to 2-mm thickness for 7 to 9 minutes. Light activation, chemical activation, or a combination of the two can be used and may be repeated as many as six times per visit, depending on the type and severity of the stain, as well as the patient's sensitivity. The curing light should be used for only 3 to 4 minutes. The gel changes from a blue-green to a cream color when oxidation is completed. For tetracycline stains, first place the gel directly on the banded areas for 3 to 4 minutes with curing-light activation as many as three times if needed. Then bleach the entire tooth through chemical oxidation.

Accel Plus 50 (Brite Smile) contains 50% hydrogen peroxide (also available in 35%) and sodium perborate. An easy-to-apply paste is formed when the ingredients are mixed together. Although the bleaching process is further accelerated through the use of heat and light, it is not necessary to use either of them to activate oxidation. This is helpful in reducing sensitivity, particularly in younger patients with larger pulp horns. This product contains flouride, calcium, and phosphate to aid in remineralization and possibly the reduction of color relapse.

Finishing

Polish all bleached teeth using the three shapes of the Shofu aluminum oxide abrasive disks and wheels (Shofu cosmetic contouring kit) (Figs 4-2n and 4-2o).

In treatments that extend over several weeks, have patients apply a 1.1% neutral sodium fluoride topical gel daily between appointments to help prevent sensitivity. A desensitization toothpaste can also be used if necessary.

After the last treatment, polish with the yellow, then the white impregnated Shofu rotary polishing wheel to achieve a high enamel luster.

Inform the patient that after bleaching the teeth initially may appear chalky white because of dehydration and that they will darken over the next few days after treatment, although to a shade lighter than the previous one. Some patients experience heightened sensitivity to cold for 1 or 2 days and should avoid cold air, drinks, and foods. Most patients are able to alleviate any discomfort in this period by taking two aspirin, acetaminophen, or nonsteroidal anti-inflammatory tablets every 4 to 6 hours. Caution patients that an annual "touch-up" bleach usually will be recommended for the removal of any new accumulated stain.

Planning for Continued Treatment

Step 14 You must use your clinical judgment to decide if continued rebleaching will provide greater improvement (Fig 4-2p to 4-2r). If the tooth shows significant improvement, then the solution chosen contained the correct solvent for the stain and rebleaching is likely to continue improvement. Conversely, if good results are not obtained, bleaching out the discoloration may not be possible.

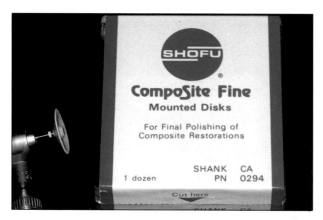

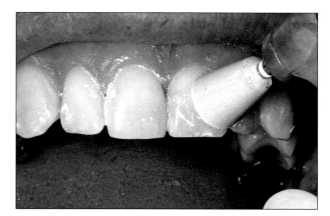

Figs 4-2n and 4-2o The teeth are polished with abrasive disks and wheels, as well as with impregnated cups.

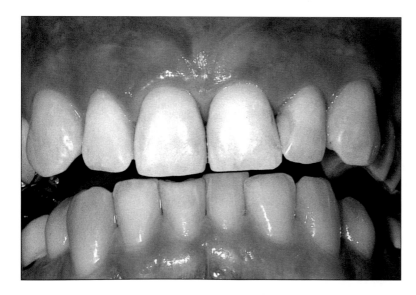

Fig 4-2p The final result shows a distinct difference between the maxillary and mandibular arches.

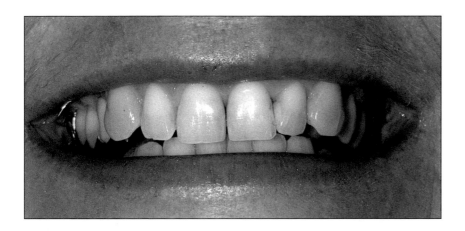

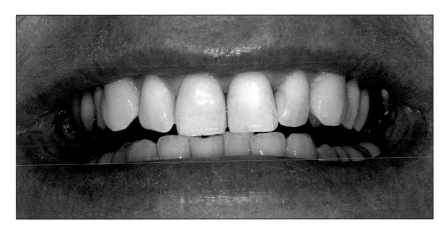

Figs 4-2q and 4-2r The main advantage of the power bleach is that it rapidly brightens the teeth in one session, which then motivates the patient to utilize several weeks of matrix therapy to maintain and enhance the color.

Bibliography

Anderson M. Dental bleaching. Curr Opin Dent 1991;1:185–191.

Dzierzak J. Factors which cause tooth color changes—protocol for in-office "power bleaching." Pract Periodont Aesthet Dent 1991;3:15–20.

Feinman RA, Goldstein RE, Garber DA. Bleaching Teeth. Chicago: Quintessence, 1987.

Goldstein RE. Bleaching teeth: new materials—new role. J Am Dent Assoc 1987;115:44E–52E.

Goldstein RE. Change Your Smile, ed 3. Chicago: Quintessence, in press.

Haywood VB. Bleaching of vital and nonvital teeth. Curr Opin Dent 1992;2:142–149.

Rada RE. Safe and effective vital tooth bleaching. CDS Review 1993;(Sep):26–30.

5

Nightguard Vital Bleaching

Harald O. Heymann, DDS, MEd
Van B. Haywood, DMD

An alternative vital bleaching technique used singularly or in combination with in-office techniques is nightguard vital bleaching. Although first reported in the dental literature by Haywood and Heymann in 1989 as "nightguard vital bleaching,"[1] this out-of-the-office technique for lightening teeth also has been referred to as home bleaching, matrix bleaching, mouthguard bleaching, and dentist-prescribed/home-applied bleaching.[2-7] Regardless of the terminology, this is a simple, apparently safe, and comparatively inexpensive bleaching alternative for patients.

The technique involves the application of a mild bleaching agent to the teeth through the wearing of a custom-made, vacuum-formed appliance (Fig 5-1). The bleaching agent typically employed is 10% to 15% carbamide peroxide, also termed hydrogen peroxide carbamide, carbamide urea, urea peroxide, or perhydrol urea.[8] Upon exposure to oral fluids, 10% carbamide peroxide has been shown to break down during oxidation into its constituent parts—water, urea, and oxygen—which appear to be safely handled by the body. Ten percent carbamide peroxide is equivalent in strength to 3% hydrogen peroxide. This concentration is considerably milder than the 30% to 35% hydrogen peroxide generally used for in-office vital bleaching ("power bleaching")

> *The bleaching process proceeds more rapidly if daytime wear of the nightguard is employed in combination with nighttime wear, compared to nighttime use only.*

techniques. However, because of the lower comparative strength of the bleaching agent, considerably more time is required to achieve comparable bleaching results. Typically, nightguard vital bleaching will attain optimal lightening in approximately 2 to 6 weeks. The rapidity with which the final results are obtained depends primarily upon the daily treatment or exposure times and the degree of discoloration present in the teeth. Bleaching results are dose/time-related. The greater the exposure time for a given concentration, the faster the final results are obtained. Consequently, the bleaching process proceeds more rapidly if daytime wear of the nightguard is employed in combination with nighttime wear, compared to daytime or nighttime use only.

Most current bleaching preparations intended for nightguard use contain a synthetic polymer thickening agent, Carbopol (B. F. Goodrich), which renders the material more thixotropic, resulting in better retention in the nightguard. The addition of Carbopol also slows the rate of oxygen release, extending the duration of the bleaching action. This oxidation-retarding effect makes Carbopol-containing bleaching agents preferred, especially for nighttime use.[9] Daytime use typically consists of 1- to 2-hour applications one to two times a day.

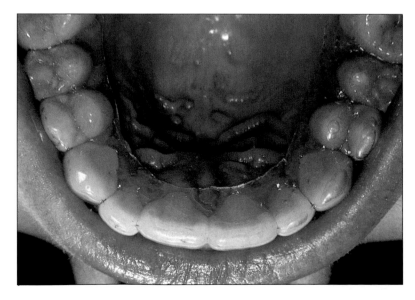

Fig 5-1 Example of shape and fit of the custom-fitted nightguard with the bleaching solution inserted.

As with all vital bleaching techniques, results are not totally predictable. However, according to a study conducted by Clinical Research Associates under the direction of Dr Gordon Christensen, 7,617 dentists surveyed indicated a success rate of greater than 90% with the nightguard vital bleaching technique.[10] Ninety percent of the responding dentists noted using 10% carbamide peroxide as the bleaching agent. These results are consistent with those noted in a more controlled clinical study conducted at the University of North Carolina. In this study, 92% of the patients experienced some lightening of their teeth after 6 weeks.[11] This color was maintained for 2 to 3 years with no further treatment.

Although predictable outcomes are not absolute, nightguard vital bleaching appears to offer consistently effective results when case selection is optimally determined. It also should be noted that when used together in combination, in-office and nightguard vital bleaching techniques often achieve superior results to those obtained through the use of either approach alone.

History

As noted earlier, nightguard vital bleaching was first reported in the dental literature by Haywood and Heymann in 1989. However, the technique actually originated over 20 years earlier. As with many notable discoveries, the nightguard vital bleaching technique was discovered largely by accident.[12,13]

Dr Bill Klusmier, an orthodontist in Fort Smith, Arkansas, was completing treatment of a patient who sustained trauma to the mouth. The patient was in the retention phase of the orthodontic treatment and periodically was wearing an orthodontic positioner (similar to a custom-fitted nightguard). In an effort to facilitate tissue healing, Dr Klusmier instructed his patient to place an over-the-counter oral antiseptic, Gly-oxide (Marion Merell Dow), containing 10% carbamide peroxide into the orthodontic positioner at night. Dr Klusmier noted a significant improvement in tissue health, but more importantly, discovered that the patient also returned with lighter teeth after an extended period of time. He began using this technique for bleaching teeth.

Upon the introduction of Proxigel (Reed and Carnrick), Dr Klusmier switched to this over-the-counter oral antiseptic because of its thixotropic consistency, which allowed it to be better retained in the appliance. He subsequently proceeded to use a custom-fitted nightguard solely for the purpose of bleaching. Dr Klusmier presented his findings from 1970 to 1975 at several dental meetings, including the Arkansas State Dental Society Meeting, and shared his findings with some of his colleagues.

One such colleague was Dr Jerry Wagner, a pediatric dentist who also practiced in Fort Smith and who was a fellow member of a local study club to which Dr Klusmier belonged. While treating some older children with minor orthodontics, Dr Wagner noted similar problems with gingival inflammation associated with poor oral hygiene. Consequently, he also directed patients to place Proxigel in a custom-fitted mouthguard to help improve tissue health. At recalls, not only was improved tissue health evident, but also a concomitant lightening of the teeth was noted. Consequently, he too began offering this esthetic treatment as an optional service to patients desiring lighter teeth.

The technique spread by word of mouth among a number of practitioners. In 1984, Dr Wagner shared the technique with Dr Tom Austin, a general dentist from North Carolina who successfully used the technique on family members and subsequently on patients. A year later, he in turn conveyed the technique to Dr David Freshwater, a fellow North Carolina dentist who presented the technique to his local study club, the Coastal Dental Study Club. The members of this study club used this nightguard vital bleaching technique frequently and shared the technique with Dr Haywood of the University of North Carolina in April 1988, while he was presenting a continuing education course to this study group.

After returning to the University of North Carolina, Drs Haywood and Heymann began clinical and laboratory investigations of the technique, which precipitated the publication of the first article on this technique.

In 1986, a parallel discovery of the lightening capabilities of a 10% carbamide peroxide solution was made by Dr John Munro, a general dentist in Tennessee. Dr Munro originally was using 10% carbamide peroxide (Gly-oxide) to treat gingival tissues following periodontal root planing. The antiseptic solution often was placed in a vacuum-formed plastic splint to facilitate application of the material to the periodontal site. Patients were instructed to replace the solution periodically to enhance treatment efficacy. He, too, noticed the lightening effects of the carbamide peroxide as a side effect of the treatment.

Dr Munro shared his findings in 1988 with a dental manufacturer, Omnii International, which subsequently developed and in 1989 marketed White and Brite, the first commercially available 10% carbamide peroxide bleaching solution intended for use with a custom-fabricated nightguard.[2]

Since that time, many bleaching preparations have appeared on the market, including some marketed directly to the public for use without dentist supervision.[14] Unfortunately these "quick fix" bleaching products marketed to the public often contained fairly acidic conditioners or prerinsing agents that could potentially harm tooth structure if used over extended periods.[7,15] In many cases, the efficacy of these products was also suspect. In response to these unsupervised bleaching regimens and to the rapid uncontrolled proliferation of the many new bleaching products, in 1991 the FDA issued a statement to manufacturers requiring the submission of appropriate documentation of safety and efficacy prior to marketing these products.[16] This action did not restrict the dentist's ability to continue nightguard vital bleaching techniques for patients, but rather protected consumers against products that were potentially harmful and, in some cases, fraudulent. This action was later rescinded when challenged by a dental manufacturer. The American Dental Association has subsequently developed guidelines for receiving ADA acceptance.[17] Nightguard vital bleaching techniques with products containing 10% to 15% carbamide peroxide appear to be safe and effective, but nonetheless, should always be administered with known products from reputable manufacturers and only under the supervision of a dentist.[7,8]

> *Nightguard vital bleaching techniques with products containing 10% to 15% carbamide peroxide appear to be safe and effective.*

Indications and Contraindications

As with other vital bleaching techniques, nightguard vital bleaching achieves the best results for patients in whom the teeth are yellow, orange, or light musky brown in coloration (Figs 5-2a and 5-2b). Teeth with dark blue-gray staining due to a past history of tetracycline administration do not typically respond well to this technique. Nonetheless, some lightening of tetracycline-stained teeth can be achieved with extended treatment times, especially if combined with in-office bleaching treatments (Figs 5-3a and 5-3b).

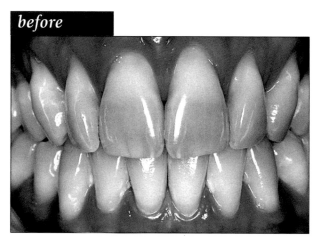
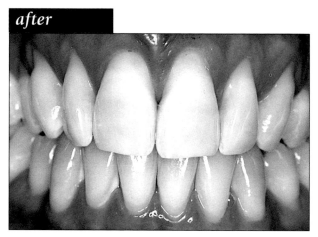

Figs 5-2a and 5-2b Typical before and after photographs of teeth successfully bleached with nightguard vital bleaching.

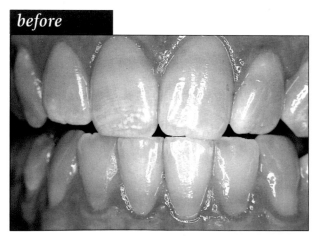
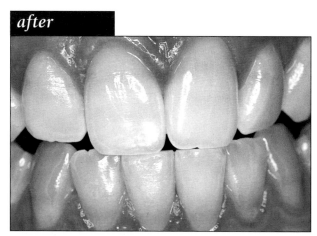

Figs 5-3a and 5-3b Before and after photographs of tetracycline-stained teeth bleached with nightguard vital bleaching.

Another indication for the use of nightguard vital bleaching is for the treatment of brown fluorosis stains (Figs 5-4a and 5-4b). Brownish discolored areas resulting from this etiologic factor respond quite well to this treatment. However, the white opaque areas often found in conjunction with brown fluorosis stains are not resolved. Typically, these "white spots" become less apparent with bleaching of the tooth in this manner, because the surrounding tooth structure lightens, making the white spots less evident.

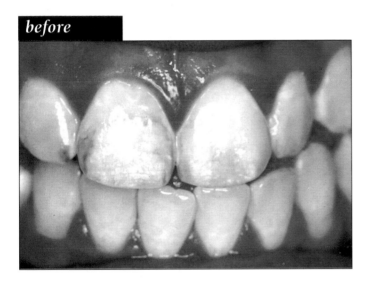

before

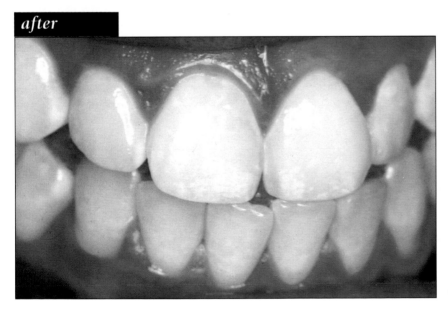

after

Figs 5-4a and 5-4b Brown fluorosis stains before and after treatment with nightguard vital bleaching.

Although multiple discolored anterior teeth are treated most easily with this technique, single discolored anterior teeth may be treated as well (Figs 5-5a and 5-5b). If the patient does not wish to lighten all the anterior teeth, the nightguard or bleaching matrix itself may be modified to facilitate bleaching a single tooth. Fabrication of this modified nightguard is described later. Extended bleaching times also may be required to resolve significant yellow discoloration of single vital anterior teeth, especially if the staining is associated with a history of trauma and calcific metamorphosis of the pulp chamber is evident.

before

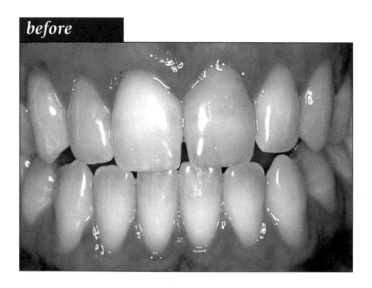

after

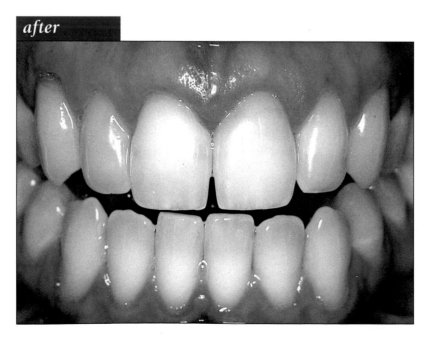

Figs 5-5a and 5-5b Single dark tooth treated without altering the color of the adjacent teeth.

Single anterior teeth that are significantly more discolored may also be treated in conjunction with treatment of all the anterior teeth (Figs 5-6a and 5-6b). The bleaching treatment for the single more discolored tooth is simply extended beyond the time it takes to lighten the other anterior teeth. Once the anterior teeth have been lightened, the remaining darker tooth is bleached by placing the bleaching agent in the single space in the nightguard corresponding to this darker tooth. The adjacent teeth will not be affected by further exposure to the bleaching agent if they already have been optimally lightened.

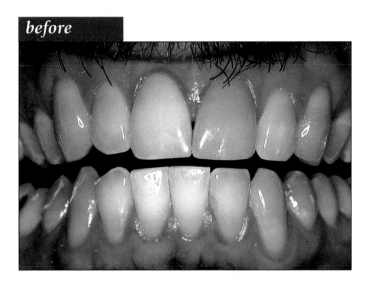

before

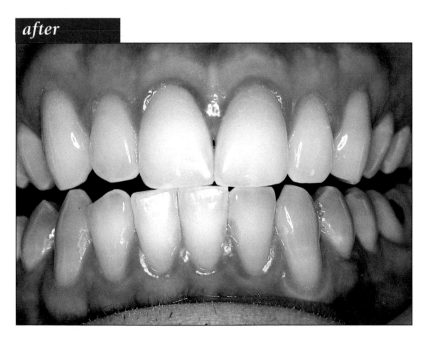

after

Figs 5-6a and 5-6b Single dark tooth lightened in conjunction with bleaching of all maxillary anterior teeth to achieve a more harmonious shade. Also note shade change, especially in the canines.

Nightguard vital bleaching techniques, used singularly or in conjunction with conventional in-office bleaching, can also be most useful in restoring teeth to their lighter coloration following years of exposure to the staining influences of smoking, coffee, tea, and/or other chromogenic foods. Teeth that have darkened in this manner often no longer match adjacent or opposing crowns or other prostheses. This mismatch in color significantly compromises dental esthetics and is frequently considered unsightly by the patient. By bleaching the natural unrestored teeth, the original shade often can be achieved and a match with other existing prostheses obtained (Figs 5-7a and 5-7b). Through this very conservative approach, nightguard vital bleaching can frequently reverse the staining effects associated with the aging process and restore a color match with existing restorations.

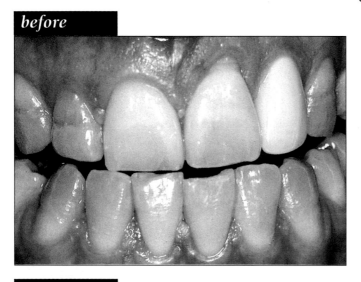

before

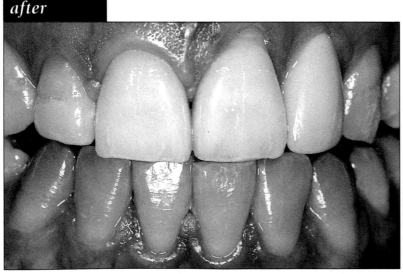

after

Figs 5-7a and 5-7b Single porcelain-fused-to-metal crown that originally blended with dentition, but which no longer matches anterior teeth due to their age-related discoloration. Lightening natural teeth to match the crown's original shade lengthens the life of the restoration.

This same approach also can be used to salvage an existing anterior prosthesis that is simply too light in shade. Due to economic considerations, many patients cannot afford to replace an existing crown or bridge that, when placed, was too light in shade. Assuming the fit, contour, and occlusal relationship of the prosthesis are otherwise acceptable, the adjacent teeth often can be bleached sufficiently to achieve acceptable esthetics, saving the patient considerable time and expense. It should be noted, however, that ordinarily all bleaching should be performed prior to the placement of any anticipated anterior restorations or prostheses (Figs 5-8a and 5-8b). However, ample time always should be allowed after the bleaching treatment for the bleached teeth to "stabilize" in color prior to pursuing any esthetic restorative treatment.

before

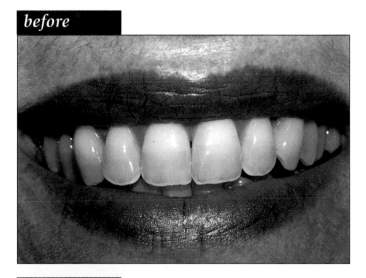

after

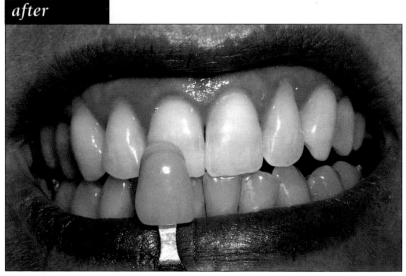

Figs 5-8a and 5-8b Without preoperative bleaching, teeth of this discoloration would present a restorative challenge should restorations or crowns be indicated.

An interesting future indication for nightguard vital bleaching appears to be in the reduction of the staining associated with chlorhexidine treatments. Pilot clinical studies at the University of North Carolina have demonstrated a significant decrease in the dark staining characteristic of chlorhexidine treatment when 10% carbamide peroxide is used in an alternating application with the chlorhexidine mouthwash. Later reports support this concept.[18]

Because of the anticariogenic characteristics of carbamide peroxide, custom-made mouthguards or matrices are being examined for the application of this medicament to effect a reduction in root surface caries.[19] Use of this system also is being considered for the treatment of the gingival inflammation associated with gingivitis and acute necrotizing ulcerative gingivitis (ANUG). However, no definitive conclusions can yet be made regarding either of these potential uses. The lightening of discolored teeth far and away remains the primary application of the nightguard vital bleaching technique.

Some concern still exists regarding the indications or contraindications for bleaching teeth with existing cervical abrasion or erosion lesions. Nightguard vital bleaching is generally not a problem when bleaching teeth with exposed root surfaces or cervical eroded areas, as long as these areas are not hypersensitive. Hypersensitive teeth are best treated first with a desensitizing agent, such as those that deposit calcium oxalate crystals in the dentinal tubules. Desensitizing toothpastes containing fluoride or sodium nitrate also may be used. Exposed dentinal surfaces in cervical areas are otherwise not at significant risk when using nightguard vital bleaching techniques, because studies show that the peroxide component passes freely through tooth structure regardless. The low molecular weight of the peroxide molecule allows free passage through both enamel and dentin. For this same reason, little concern exists when bleaching teeth with existing potentially "leaky" restorations. These restorations need not be replaced prior to nightguard vital bleaching.

Finally, although nightguard vital bleaching appears to be most safe and effective under normal use, it is not recommended in heavy smokers or users of tobacco products, unless they are willing to refrain from tobacco use during treatment. Although no conclusive evidence is available, studies do suggest that the carcinogenic effects of DMBA, a known carcinogen associated with tobacco products, may be elevated in the presence of oxygenating agents.[20] Furthermore, as is prudent policy for most drugs, the administration of nightguard vital bleaching agents is not recommended in pregnant or lactating women.

Bleaching Agents

As noted earlier, the most predominantly used material for nightguard vital bleaching is carbamide peroxide. Historically, this material has been used as an oral antiseptic for the treatment of minor oral irritations or inflammation.[21] In fact, 10% to 15% carbamide peroxide, along with 1.5% and 3% hydrogen peroxide, are classified as "oral antiseptics" by the US Food and Drug Administration (FDA) in the FDA monograph of 1988. According to this publication, these concentrations of carbamide peroxide and hydrogen peroxide are classified as "Category I" materials, which are "generally recognized as safe and effective and not misbranded."[22]

Carbamide peroxide in a concentration of 10% to 15% is today typically used in most nightguard vital beaching agents. However, a significant difference in these materials lies in the presence or absence of carboxymethylene polymer or Carbopol 940 (B. F. Goodrich). This material originated as a unique ingredient incorporated in the now-expired patent for Proxigel (Reed and Carnrick). According to the patent, the purpose of the incorporation of Carbopol in Proxigel was to "thicken the material, improve tissue adherence, and prolong the release of oxygen" when compared to its precursor in the oral antiseptic market, Gly-oxide (Marion Merell Dow).[23] These characteristics also made the incorporation of Carbopol a logical addition to most other nightguard vital bleaching agents.

Based on this distinction, virtually all existing carbamide peroxide–containing nightguard vital bleaching agents can be divided into solutions containing Carbopol and solutions without Carbopol. It should be noted that Carbopol-containing solutions require less frequent replenishment in the nightguard due to slower oxygen release owing to the presence of the Carbopol. This quality, plus the more thixotropic nature of the Carbopol-containing bleaching materials, makes them ideal for nightguard vital bleaching applications. Recently, some products have introduced non-Carbopol thickeners. Since the additives do not necessarily retard oxygen release, they are generally applied for 1 to 2 hours, once or twice a day. [24]

Clinical Technique

Nightguard vital bleaching generally requires only an initial consultation appointment, a nightguard delivery appointment, and brief periodic visits to monitor patient progress during the course of treatment. Collectively, these appointments require minimal in-office chairtime.[25]

At the first consultation appointment, the patient's medical history and dental history are reviewed or taken. Appropriate radiographs are reviewed or made. If the patient is not already a patient of record, an intraoral examination of the teeth to be bleached, soft tissues, periodontal health, and the occlusal relationship of the teeth also should be performed at a minimum. A complete examination and charting is recommended if additional dental treatment is indicated.

At this first appointment, a complete description of the nightguard vital bleaching technique should be given to the patient, as well as a review of any potential problems, side effects, or sequelae.[26] If the dentist prefers, much of this information can be sent to the patient prior to the consultation appointment. This approach allows the patient to formulate questions and allows the dentist to better spend his or her time during the consultation appointment examining the patient and responding to questions. In any case, it is recommended to provide a written copy of this information to the patient, which can also serve as a notice of informed consent. The patient also must be informed that existing anterior restorations that match the existing pretreatment shade of the teeth may require partial or total replacement following the bleaching treatment, since they often no longer will match the lighter shade of the teeth. This point is of particular importance, since the cost of replacing these restorations may, in fact, exceed the cost of the bleaching treatment.

Photographs of similar cases before and after treatment are invaluable for showing patients the types of results that can be expected. In these photographs, it is desirable to have only one arch bleached so the opposite arch can be used for comparison. Computer imaging also can be used to help the patient visualize what the final outcome may look like. However, it must be emphasized that the results are not totally predictable and are subject to variation among individuals. Therefore, imaging must be viewed as a "best guess" or simulation only. As previously noted, many imaging systems allow the inclusion of a disclaimer directly on the printout.

A shade determination should then be made of the teeth to be bleached with a Vita or comparable shade guide. This information is recorded in the chart as a baseline for future reference. By comparing the postoperative shade to this pretreatment shade, the degree of tooth lightening can readily be determined. Preoperative photographs are recommended, as they represent the best form of documentation for future reference. In addition to photographing the teeth alone, photographs also should be made including the appropriate shade tab positioned in the photographic field as a constant standard for comparison.

> *It must be emphasized that the results are not totally predictable and are subject to variation among individuals.*

It is highly recommended that the teeth be bleached in one arch at a time, beginning with the maxillary arch. There are several reasons for this. First, the maxillary arch typically bleaches faster than the mandibular arch. This observation is attributed to better retention of the bleaching agent in the maxillary nightguard, due both to gravity and to reduced effects from salivary flow compared to the mandibular arch. Second, by bleaching the maxillary arch first, the mandibular arch is maintained as a constant comparative standard for the continual monitoring of bleaching efficacy. Third, bleaching both arches simultaneously interposes two thicknesses of nightguard material, which may contribute to occlusal or TMJ problems. And, finally, if bleaching in the maxillary arch is unsuccessful, the time and expense of needlessly bleaching the mandibular arch is saved.

As the last part of this first appointment, an alginate impression is made of the maxillary arch from which a hydrocal (dental stone) cast is generated. This cast is required for subsequent fabrication of a vacuum-formed nightguard. This process is described on pages 90 to 92.

The second appointment is the nightguard delivery appointment. Before the actual try-in, the nightguard should be examined closely for internal positive blebs that could act as pressure points in the nightguard, and for rough peripheral edges. The finished nightguard is trial-positioned in the patient's mouth and closely evaluated for overall fit, tissue adaptation, and retention. Peripheral edges of the nightguard also must be examined closely in the mouth by both the dentist and the patient to identify potentially irritating areas. The edges must be smooth and regular in outline form. The tissue may be viewed through the nightguard to evaluate for blanching. Patients should practice inserting and removing the guard, being careful not to traumatize the gingiva with their fingernails in the canine region. The nightguard is best removed by "peeling" the material from the posterior section beginning on one side of the arch.

After the fit of the nightguard is determined to be satisfactory, the occlusion should be evaluated, with the patient closing his or her teeth together. Generally, the thinness of the material allows reasonable contact of all the teeth in maximum intercuspation. However, the thinness of the nightguard precludes adjustment of the occlusion. If premature contacts exist on the terminal molar teeth upon closure, the nightguard must be trimmed to remove this terminal molar area until the occlusal relationship of the teeth with the nightguard in place is satisfactory. It is not advisable to prophylactically remove the terminal portion of the nightguard unless occlusion or comfort dictates the necessity. Also, it is recommended that the patient be consulted or advised prior to removing the terminal molar area from the nightguard to understand the necessity of the action. As odd as it seems, some patients insist on bleaching all of their teeth, even if the teeth cannot be seen!

Proper insertion of the carbamide peroxide material into the nightguard and positioning of the nightguard over the teeth should be reviewed with the patient. There is no known harm if patients swallow the solution, but they should be warned prior to inserting the guard that the taste may be somewhat "like medicine." If the taste is particularly unpleasant, either a cotton swab dipped in mouthwash and applied to the posterior portion of the tongue after insertion or construction of a nightguard that covers the palate can reduce this annoyance. Patients should not rinse their mouth once the nightguard is inserted unless the manufacturer's instructions specify it. Provide the patient with a plastic orthodontic retainer box for storage of the nightguard when not in use.

Information regarding nightguard vital bleaching, including potential problems or side effects, should again be reviewed with the patient. Specific patient instructions for use of the nightguard vital bleaching technique also should be included with this information.

Two primary treatment regimens are presented for nightguard vital bleaching: nighttime application and daytime use. For

> *The rapidity with which final results are achieved is based largely on the total exposure time of the teeth to the bleaching agent, regardless of the regimen employed.*

patients that do not wish to wear the nightguard during the daytime, instructions for nighttime use are provided. If worn only at night, bleaching usually requires a period of 2 to 6 weeks for optimal results. Darkly stained teeth may warrant even longer treatment. If a daytime approach is opted for or combined with nighttime wear, final results can be achieved in as little as 1½ to 2 weeks.

No one treatment regimen is deemed the best. The choice of a specific treatment option is primarily based on patient preferences and the incidence of side effects. The rapidity with which final results are achieved is based largely on the total exposure time of the teeth to the bleaching agent, regardless of the regimen employed. However, if the patient elects to pursue a daytime or combination daytime/nighttime schedule, it is recommended that the patient begin the bleaching process slowly and gradually increase the exposure time as the treatment progresses. By titrating the exposure time, tolerance to the bleaching agent is improved and fewer side effects are noted. The general patient instructions for Carbopol-containing bleaching materials are as follows:

Patient Instructions

Nighttime Schedule

1. Brush and floss your teeth prior to bedtime.
2. Place 2 to 3 drops or a thin bead of the carbamide peroxide bleaching material into the space of the nightguard corresponding to each tooth to be bleached.
3. Insert the nightguard in the mouth over the teeth. Expectorate the excess bleaching material. Some materials may require wiping excess from tissue with a finger or clean toothbrush, or rinsing with water.
4. Wear the loaded nightguard during the night and remove it in the morning. Wipe or rinse material from the teeth. Aggressive brushing is not indicated or desirable.[27]
5. Clean the nightguard with a toothbrush. Rinse, dry, and store in the retainer box provided for storage of the nightguard.

Daytime Schedule

1. Place 2 to 3 drops or a thin bead of the carbamide peroxide bleaching material into the space of the nightguard corresponding to each tooth to be bleached.
2. Insert the nightguard in the mouth over the teeth. Expectorate the excess bleaching material. Remove excess material from the gingiva by wiping with a finger or a toothbrush.
3. Replenish the carbamide peroxide bleaching material after 1 to 2 hours, or according to the manufacturer's instructions. Repeat applications are possible; however, do not exceed a total wearing time (including any nighttime wear) of approximately 12 hours per day to allow adequate time for tissue recuperation and occlusal stabilization.
4. Do not wear the nightguard during meals. Use normal oral hygiene procedures prior to the insertion of the loaded nightguard.
5. Clean the nightguard after use with a toothbrush. Rinse, dry, and store it in the retainer box provided for nightguard storage.

All patient instructions also should note that minor sensitivity to cold may be encountered. However, patient instructions also should emphasize that wearing of the nightguard should be discontinued if the nightguard is uncomfortable, if soft tissue irritations occur, or if tooth sensitivity is severe. Most treatment sequelae are related to problems with the nightguard. Side effects due to the bleaching agent itself are usually mild, transient, and dose-related.[11] Reducing the exposure time or temporarily discontinuing treatment generally alleviates these problems. Although true allergies to the bleaching agent are rare, bleaching treatment should be discontinued if soft tissue reactions suggest that an allergy exists. It is important to note that clinical studies reveal that none of the side effects persist upon termination of treatment.[10,11]

Patients also should be informed that the teeth may appear "splotchy" during the early stages of treatment due to differences in the coverage of the tooth with the bleaching agent or differences in response by the tooth. However, patients should be assured that a more homogeneous appearance can be expected with continued treatment.

All patients should be recalled periodically during nightguard vital bleaching. Most potential postoperative problems will emerge within the first week of treatment. The frequency of patient recall appointments is determined based on the treatment regimen and patient response. Patients using a nighttime schedule of bleaching may require longer recall intervals due to the longer treatment time.

Once it has been determined that optimal lightening of the teeth has been obtained, treatment should be discontinued. Some dentists prefer retaining the nightguard to prevent unauthorized and uncontrolled bleaching by the patient, while others give this responsibility to the patient. Regardless, the patient must be made to understand that nightguard vital bleaching should be undertaken only while under the supervision of a dentist. A final shade assessment should be made and recorded in the patient's chart for future reference in determining the need for retreatment. Postoperative photographs should also be taken at this time, including those in which the shade tab is positioned in the photographic field. Treatment of the mandibular arch, if desired, is accomplished in the same way as the maxillary arch.

Nightguard Fabrication

An alginate impression (Jeltrate Plus, L. D. Caulk) is made of the arch to be bleached as noted earlier. The impression is rinsed under running water and sprayed with glutaraldehyde (OMNI II, Omni-Tech Medical) for infection control. It is rinsed, then sprayed again. After at least 3 minutes exposure to the glutaraldehyde, the impression can be handled safely with ungloved hands. The impression is then washed vigorously under running water to avoid the disinfectant inhibiting the set of the hydrocal (dental stone). Failure to adequately rinse the impression of the disinfectant will result in a cast with a softened surface that is easily abraded. This softened surface can result in the fabrication of a nightguard that is too small in certain areas. A nightguard that is too small can result in two common side effects: *(1)* gingival irritation and *(2)* tooth soreness.

The disinfected, rinsed impression is poured with hydrocal. The resultant cast must be free of voids, significant blebs (positives), and chips. The cast is trimmed on a model trimmer to achieve a base parallel to the occlusal plane of the posterior teeth, and to eliminate the land area beyond the depth of the vestibule. The base of the cast should be flat and either very thin or with a hole in the center. Ideally, the cast should be allowed to dry at least 24 hours prior to nightguard fabrication. Some fast-setting stones allow fabrication of the nightguard in one visit. Minor voids and significant undercuts can be blocked out with clay or a puttylike material (Block-out Compound, Buffalo Manufacturing) prior to fabrication of the nightguard. Wax should not be used, as it will melt during the fabrication process. Failure to block out voids can result in positives in the nightguard, which can cause undesirable minor orthodontic forces being exerted on teeth. This often results in tooth discomfort.

Some of the more highly viscous bleaching materials may require the establishment of a reservoir on the facial aspect of each tooth. These reservoirs are formed by the addition of light-cured composite spacers or similar materials to the cast. The reservoirs allow for easier seating of the nightguard when using a highly viscous bleaching material. Although clinically nightguard adaptation decreases with reservoirs present, the use of the highly viscous material compensates for decreased retention of the nightguard. Reservoirs are generally *not* recommended for most 10% to 15% carbamide peroxide bleaching agents containing Carbopol with viscosities similar to that of Proxigel.

Another tray design employs the use of a foam spacer between the teeth and the guard. However, the use of the spacer has not been shown in clinical trials to shorten the treatment time or improve the efficacy of the bleaching treatment.[28] Use of the foam spacer also compromises the esthetics and has a greater impact on the occlusion.

A heat/vacuum tray-forming machine (Sta-Vac, Buffalo Manufacturing) is used to fabricate the nightguard. The machine needs to warm up for 10 minutes prior to fabrication of the nightguard to ensure uniform heating of the material. The nightguard may be fabricated using a .020" material (#31720 coping material, Buffalo Manufacturing) or a .035" material (Opalescence Softray, Ultradent). These thinner materials allow construction of a nightguard with minimal effects on occlusion, esthetics, and phonetics. Upon softening to the point that the material sags about one inch, the vacuum is engaged, and the heated nightguard material lowered slowly onto the cast to avoid generating wrinkles or folds in the material. Ample time under vacuum must be allowed for the material to be well-adapted to the cast. Premature cessation of the vacuum will result in a poorly defined and inadequately retentive nightguard. The nightguard should be allowed to cool on the cast prior to furthur manipulation.

The nightguard is trimmed while still on the cast using a #12 surgical blade in a Bard-Parker handle. Care must be taken to avoid injury. Another option is to use a bur in a slow-speed handpiece. Scribe a continuous line approximately 3 mm beyond the teeth, creating a horseshoe design. Remove the excess outer portion of the nightguard material first, including the inner portion corresponding to the palatal or tongue space. The resulting horseshoe-shaped nightguard is then removed from the cast. Sharp, curved, nonserrated scissors can be used to trim and refine the periphery of the nightguard. The edge of the nightguard may extend approximately 2 mm from the gingival crest onto the gingival tissue. Trimming of the periphery should allow for frenum attachments and their unrestricted movement. The nightguard should not extend into any tissue undercuts, and the incisal papilla should not be covered, if possible. If it is not possible to trim the nightguard to exclude the incisal papilla, then the border of the nightguard should be terminated in an area between rugae of the hard palate to avoid irritation of the tongue. One manufacturer's material requires special serrated scissors (supplied by the manufacturer) for smoothest trimming. Initially, the nightguard can extend onto the gingival tissue as previously described. However, should the patient experience tissue discomfort, the nightguard can be either shortened to avoid coverage of the particular area or trimmed in a scalloped fashion to follow the contours of the tissue, so that only the teeth are covered by the nightguard.

If the patient only has one tooth that is darkened and is satisfied with the color of the other teeth, a single-tooth non-scalloped bleaching nightguard may be constructed. The technique for nightguard fabrication is the same as previously described, except that after completion of the nightguard, a "window" is trimmed on either side of the tooth to be lightened (Fig 5-9). As noted earlier, bleaching solution then is placed only in the single-tooth portion of the nightguard. Excess material will be extruded through the adjacent spaces created by the window.

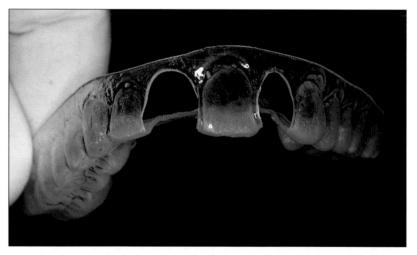

Fig 5-9 Example of nightguard with "window design" for bleaching a single tooth.

Safety Issues and Current Research

Because of the simplicity and ease of nightguard vital bleaching, there has been rapid acceptance of the technique by dentists. Nonetheless, concerns exist regarding the safety and efficacy of these materials and this technique.

A 10% solution of carbamide peroxide is composed of 3% hydrogen peroxide and 7% urea. The hydrogen peroxide breaks down into water and oxygen, while the urea breaks down into carbon dioxide and ammonia. All four products are easily handled by the normal body processes. Hydrogen peroxide is a normally occurring body component, and is scavenged by enzymes called peroxidases. Urea is also a normal body component found in saliva, which tends to raise salivary pH. Hydrogen peroxide is found in plant foods, air, and water, and is used to prepare foods and drinks. It is generally recognized as safe as a food ingredient when certain limitations are imposed.[29]

The two primary side effects that may occur during treatment are a transient sensitivity of the teeth to cold and irritation of the gingiva. Approximately two-thirds of patients undergoing treatment will experience one or both of these side effects.[11] However, the majority of these side effects are of 1 to 4 days in duration, and all side effects cease upon termination of treatment as noted earlier, with no long-term effects noted.[11]

Tooth sensitivity is not related to age, exposed root surface or dentin, caries, or pulp size, but rather to the easy passage of hydrogen peroxide through enamel and dentin to the pulp due to its small molecular size.[8] Treatment for sensitivity may consist of removal of the nightguard for 2 to 3 days, reduction of wearing time, or a new nightguard fabricated from a new impression if the nightguard is determined to be too small or inaccurately fitted.

Gingival irritation is related to either the fit of the nightguard or the bleaching solution itself. Inspection of the internal aspect of the nightguard for positives and viewing through the guard for tissue blanching are important. The edges of the nightguard also should be inspected for rough areas that may irritate the tissue. Shortening or smoothing the borders of the nightguard or making a new impression and nightguard generally will resolve the mechanical irritation. Reduction of wearing time or cessation of treatment for 2 to 3 days usually will allow the tissue to better accommodate the bleaching agent.

Initial safety concerns regarding the teeth surrounded issues of pH perceived to be acidic for the bleaching solutions. Since the caries process starts when the pH is below 5.5 for enamel[30] and 6.0 for dentin,[31] there was concern that the teeth would be more susceptible to caries during the bleaching process. Later research has indicated that carbamide peroxide in the pH range from 5.3 to 7.2 does not cause any perceptible etching of the teeth.[32,33] It also has been demonstrated that there is no appreciable subsurface softening of the enamel from applications of carbamide peroxide bleaching solutions, other than slight clinically insignificant changes in the first 25 µm for the lower-pH solutions.[27]

> *There is no appreciable subsurface softening of the enamel from applications of carbamide peroxide bleaching solutions.*

Generally, the effects of carbamide peroxide bleaching are considered no worse than those resulting from routinely used commercial soft drinks or other dental procedures.[7]

Due to the presence of urea (a breakdown product of the carbamide peroxide bleaching solution), the salivary pH is elevated for the first 2 hours after insertion of the nightguard.[34] The pH of the material in the nightguard elevates in 5 minutes and remains well above neutral for at least 2 hours. These factors minimize pH concerns.

No evidence of pulpal damage from carbamide peroxide has been shown.[8] As mentioned earlier, the sensitivity of the teeth is due to the easy passage of the hydrogen peroxide and urea through the enamel and dentin to the pulp. As with 35% hydrogen peroxide bleaching preparations, this tooth sensitivity is probably due to a reversible pulpitis. Much research has been conducted regarding the effects of 35% hydrogen peroxide solutions in conjunction with heat or light on pulpal response. The results of these tests are that any damage to the pulp is either nonexistent or reversible after 2 months.[35,36] The effects on the pulp of the 10% carbamide peroxide, which is effectively 3% hydrogen peroxide, would be expected to be even less.[37]

No major effects on restorative materials have been noted, although there is some concern regarding existing composite restorations. Some in vitro studies suggest the potential for shortening the effective life of a posterior composite due to softening or cracking of the resin matrix.[38] However, these studies also note that the effects of the bleaching solutions in vivo may be no worse than those of other foodstuffs. Composite resins do not appear to change color, although there may be a cleansing of both the margins and the surface of the restoration. If there is any change in the color of composite resins, it is usually clinically insignificant relative to the overall change in tooth color. Patients must be prepared to replace any esthetic restorations if the post-treatment color match is not satisfactory.

Another safety concern regarding nightguard vital bleaching is the potential for hydrogen peroxide, the breakdown product of carbamide peroxide, to cause soft tissue changes promoting cancer. Although concerns exist in the literature regarding this issue, a review of recent research on the 10% carbamide peroxide bleaching technique has not demonstrated this phenomenon.[8,39] More importantly, a review of all the research on hydrogen peroxide and its derivatives by the World Health Organization of the potential for carcinogenicity of hydrogen peroxide and other derivatives concluded that, in the absence of epidemiological data, no evaluation could be made of the carcinogenicity of hydrogen peroxide in humans.[29] Moreover, there was limited evidence of the carcinogenicity of hydrogen peroxide to experimental animals.[29] Soft tissue contact in the controlled environment of the nightguard has shown no detrimental effects. However, hydrogen peroxide has been implicated as a potentiator of known carcinogens such as those found in cigarette smoke (DMBA). Therefore, as noted earlier, patients are urged to refrain from smoking or using tobacco products during treatment.[40] The use of a scalloped tray further reduces this concern.

Carbamide peroxide has been evaluated extensively in clinical trials for uses other than bleaching teeth. It has been used in infants, adolescents, and adults for the treatment of a variety of conditions, including pharyngeal inflammations, gingival inflammation associated with orthodontic treatment, and other oral conditions.[41–49] No ill effects were reported in the results of any of these clinical studies, even though some exposure times to the carbamide peroxide significantly exceeded those associated with the nightguard vital bleaching technique.[8] Ingestion does not appear to cause any problem, other than some people do not like the taste or occasionally experience some laxative effect from the glycerine base when taken in large quantities.

Of major interest to the restorative dentist is the observation with all bleaching techniques that there is a decrease in bond strength between composite resin and bleached, etched enamel.[50] This effect also has been demonstrated with carbamide peroxide, but 1 week postbleaching the bond strengths have been shown to return to normal.[51,52] Roughening of the enamel surface also will eliminate the effects of the peroxide on bond strengths.[53] The immediate but transient reduction in bond strength is attributed to residual oxygen remaining near the enamel surface. The oxygen released inhibits the set of the bonding resin. Clinicians are advised to wait 1 to 2 weeks after cessation of any bleaching treatment before bonding composite to etched enamel.[7]

The only potential contraindication or precaution to nightguard vital bleaching is found in tetracycline-stained teeth in which one pulp chamber is markedly larger than those in the other teeth to be bleached.[54] In this situation, the affected tooth may lighten more than the other teeth. In all other bleaching situations involving teeth of dissimilar pulp sizes, the teeth with smaller pulps are either slower to lighten or do not lighten as much as the other teeth. However, with tetracycline-stained teeth, if the secondary dentin was deposited with minimal tetracycline incorporation, the tooth will seem to respond more effectively to bleaching than the other teeth. The potential outcome of having one tooth markedly lighter than the others demonstrates the importance of the preoperative radiographic examination in the initial examination appointment. Patients in this tetracycline-stained category should be aware of the potential outcome. They may still elect to proceed with bleaching treatment, because an uneven lighter color may be more preferable than the current color of their untreated tetracycline-stained teeth.

The safety and risk/benefit ratio of carbamide peroxide compare favorably to other accepted dental procedures.

The safety and risk/benefit ratio of carbamide peroxide compare favorably to other accepted dental procedures.[7] Other bleaching techniques and related research have been conducted for over 100 years. Carbamide peroxide has a long history of clinical use, both in topical intraoral tissue applications and, more recently, in tooth bleaching. There is a minimal incidence of transient side effects with nightguard vital bleaching coupled with the high percentage of success. Other color-altering treatments or actions on teeth are much more invasive and destructive. Considering these observations, it must be noted that the bleaching of vital teeth with a 10% to 15% carbamide peroxide solution containing Carbopol or another thickener administered under the supervision of a dentist using a custom-fitted nightguard is as safe as most other routinely prescribed dental treatments.

References

1. Haywood VB, Heymann HO. Nightguard vital bleaching. Quintessence Int 1989;20:173–176.
2. Darnell DH, Moore WC. Vital tooth bleaching: The White and Brite technique. Compend Contin Educ Dent 1990;11:86–94.
3. Archambault G. Caution, informed consent remain important as home bleaching grows. Dentist 1990:April:16.
4. Haywood VB. Overview and status of mouthguard bleaching. J Esthet Dent 1991;3(5):157–161.
5. Garber DA, Goldstein RE, Goldstein CE, Schwartz CG. Dentist monitored bleaching: A combined approach. Pract Periodont Aesthet Dent 1991;3(2):22–26.
6. Haywood VB. Bleaching of vital and nonvital teeth. Curr Opin Dent 1992;2:142–149.
7. Haywood VB. History, safety, and effectiveness of current bleaching techniques and applications of the nightguard vital bleaching technique. Quintessence Int 1992;23:471–488.
8. Haywood VB, Heymann HO. Nightguard vital bleaching: How safe is it? Quintessence Int 1991;22:515–523.
9. Haywood VB. Nightguard vital bleaching: current information and research. Esthet Dent Update 1990;1(2):7–12.
10. Christensen GJ. Home-use bleaching survey—1991. Clin Res Assoc Newsletter 1991;15(10):2.
11. Haywood VB, Leonard RH, Nelson CF, Brunson WD. Effectiveness, side effects and long-term status of nightguard vital bleaching. J Am Dent Assoc 1994; 125:1219–1226
12. Haywood VB. Nightguard vital bleaching: a history and products update: Part 1. Esthet Dent Update 1991;2(4):63–66.
13. Albers HF. Home bleaching. ADEPT Report 1991;2(1):9–17.
14. Stanton D. Discoveries. Dentist 1990:April;47.

15. Cubbon T, Ore D. Hard tissue and home tooth whiteners. CDS Rev 1991;85(5):32–35.

16. Berry J. FDA says whiteners are drugs. ADA News 1991;22(18):1,6,7.

17. Council on Dental Therapeutics. Guidelines for acceptance of peroxide-containing oral hygiene products. J Am Dent Assoc 1994; 125:1140–1142.

18. Sharma N, Galustians J, Curtis JP, Christina L, Jones BJB. Comparison of a carbamide peroxide in removing chlorhexidine stain [abstract 308]. J Dent Res 1995;74:50.

19. Bentley C, Broderius CA, Leonard RH, Crawford JJ. Antimicrobial effects of carbamide peroxide [abstract 1819]. J Dent Res 1995;74:239.

20. Wietzman SA, Weitberg AB, Stossel TP, et al. Effects of hydrogen peroxide on oral carcinogenesis in hamsters. J Periodontol 1986; 57:685–688.

21. Stindt DJ, Quenette L. An overview of gly-oxide liquid in control and prevention of dental disease. Compend Contin Educ Dent 1989;9:514–520.

22. Food and Drug Administration, Department of Health and Human Services. Oral health care drug products for over-the-counter human use: tentative final monograph; notice of proposed rulemaking. Fed Reg 1988;53(17):2436–2461.

23. United States Patent Office, Patent #3,657,413 April 18, 1972.

24. Haywood VB. Considerations and variations of dentist-prescribed, home-applied vital tooth bleaching techniques. Compend Contin Educ Dent 1994;15(suppl 17);s616–s621.

25. Haywood VB. Commonly asked questions about nightguard vital bleaching. Indiana Dent Assoc J 1993;72(5):28–33.

26. Haywood VB. Nightguard vital bleaching: A history and products update: Part 2. Esthet Dent Update 1991;2(5):82–85.

27. McCracken MS, Haywood VB. Effects of 10% carbamide peroxide on the subsurface hardness of enamel. Quintessence Int 1995;26;21–24.

28. Haywood VB, Leonard RH, Nelson CF. Efficacy of foam liner in 10% carbamide peroxide bleaching technique. Quintessence Int 1993;24:663–666.

29. IARC Monograph. Evaluation of carcinogenesis risk of chemicals in humans. 1985;36:285–314.

30. Schmidt-Nielsen B. The solubility of tooth substance in relation to the composition of saliva. Acta Odont Scand 1946;7(2):1–13.

31. Hoppenbrouwers PMM, Driessens FCM, Borggreven JMPM. The vulnerability of unexposed human dental roots to demineralization. J Dent Res 1986;65:955–958.

32. Haywood VB, Leech T, Heymann HO, Crumpler D, Bruggers K. Nightguard vital bleaching: effects on enamel surface texture and diffusion. Quintessence Int 1990;21:801–806.

33. Haywood VB, Houck V, Heymann HO. Nightguard vital bleaching: Effects of varying pH solutions on enamel surface texture and color change. Quintessence Int 1991;22:775–782.

34. Leonard RH, Bentley CD, Haywood VB. Salivary pH changes during 10% carbamide peroxide bleaching. Quintessence Int 1994;25:547–550.

35. Zach L, Cohen G. Pulp response to externally applied heat. Oral Surg Oral Med Oral Pathol 1965;19;515–530.

36. Nyborg H, Brannstrom M. Pulp reaction to heat. J Prosthet Dent 1968;19:605–612.

38. Bailey SJ, Swift JS Jr. Effects of home bleaching products on composite resins. Quintessence Int 1992;23:489–494.

39. Woolverton CJ, Haywood VB, Heymann HO. Toxicity of two carbamide peroxide products used in nightguard vital bleaching. Am J Dent 1993;6:310–314.

40. McCormack J. That Hollywood smile: Are tooth whiteners the answer? Access 1991;Aug:7–10.

41. Dickstein B. Neonatal oral candidiasis: Evaluation of a new chemotherapeutic agent. Clin Pediatrics 1964;3:485–488.

42. Zinner DD, Duany LF, Llorente M. Effects of urea peroxide in anhydrous glycerol on gingivitis and dental plaque. J Prevent Dent 1978;5:38–40.

43. Zinner DD, Duany LF, Chilton NW. Controlled study of the clinical effectiveness of a new oxygen gel on plaque, oral debris and gingival inflammation. Pharmacol Therapeutics Dent 1970;1:7–15.

44. Fogel MS, Magill JM. Use of an antiseptic agent in orthodontic hygiene. Dent Surv 1971;Oct:50–54.

45. Shipman B, Cohen E, Kaslick RS. The effect of a urea peroxide gel on plaque deposits and gingival status. J Periodontol 1971;42:283–285.

46. Tartakow DJ, Smith RS, Spinelli JA. Urea peroxide solution in the treatment of gingivitis in orthodontics. Am J Orthod 1978;73:560–567.

47. Williams, JC. Topical therapy for infections of the mouth and pharynx. Med Times 1963;91:332–334.

48. Shapiro WB, Kaslick RS, Chasens AI, Eisenber R. The influence of urea peroxide gel on plaque, calculus and chronic gingival inflammation. J Periodontol 1973;44:636–639.

49. Reddy J, Salkin LM. The effect of a urea peroxide rinse on dental plaque and gingivitis. J. Periodontol 1976;47:607–610.

50. Titley KC, Torneck CD, Smith DC, Adibfar A. Adhesion of composite resin to bleached and unbleached bovine enamel. J Dent Res 1988;67:1523–1528.

51. McGuckin RS, Thurmond BA, Osovitz S. In vitro enamel shear bond strengths following vital bleaching. J Dent Res 1991;70 [abstract 892]:377.

52. Torneck CD, Titley KC, Smith DC, Adibfar A. The influence of time of hydrogen peroxide exposure on the adhesion of composite resin to bleached bovine enamel. J Endodont 1990;16:123–128.

53. Cvitko E, Denehy GE, Swift EJ Jr, Pires JA. Bond strength of composite resin to enamel bleached with carbamide peroxide. J Esthet Dent 1991;3(3):100–102.

54. Haywood VB, Heymann HO. Response of normal and tetracycline-stained teeth with pulp-size variation to nightguard vital bleaching. J Esthet Dent 1994;6(3):109–114.

6

Bleaching Pulpless Teeth

David R. Steiner, DDS, MSD
John D. West, DDS, MSD

Bleaching pulpless teeth presents an esthetic challenge. This chapter describes the possibilities and pitfalls of altering the color of pulpless teeth and addresses the following questions:

1. Why do teeth discolor?
2. What are the most effective bleaching agents?
3. What is the relationship between bleaching pulpless teeth and cervical root resorption?
4. Why do teeth discolor again after bleaching?

To this end, this chapter will examine the *research* into the etiology of discoloration, discuss the relationship between bleaching and *resorption*, describe the *recipe* for predictable and safe bleaching of pulpless teeth, and present *recommendations* for successful results and troubleshooting potential problems.

Research

Why does a tooth discolor? At the clinical level, Goldstein and Feinman have divided the reasons into two broad categories: incomplete root canal therapy and pulpal degeneration.[1]

Portions of this chapter are adapted with permission from Cohen S, Burns R (eds). Pathways of the Pulp, ed 6. St Louis: Mosby, 1994.

Incomplete root canal therapy means that debris or endodontic material remains in the pulp chamber, which could cause discoloration or a change in translucency. Examples include necrotic debris in the pulp horns, filling materials located in the pulp chamber, and endodontic sealer lining the chamber walls (Figs 6-1a and 6-1b). Sealers formulated with silver powder may cause stains that are almost impossible to bleach. Special care should be taken at the time of obturation to completely remove these sealers from the chamber.

The mechanism by which pulpal degeneration causes color change is less clear. In a deeply discolored tooth, Grossman[2] attributed the darkness to iron sulfide. He hypothesized that an injury could cause bleeding into the pulp chamber. The extravasated red blood cells undergo hemolysis and release hemoglobin. Iron in the hemoglobin combines with hydrogen sulfide produced by bacteria to form iron sulfide, a very dark pigment (Figs 6-2a and 6-2b). However, the degree of discoloration of some teeth is more subtle. Is there a difference in the biochemistry of the two situations, or is it just a matter of degree? A search of dental literature and interviews with research biochemists leaves that question unanswered. Knowing the precise biochemical nature of discoloration would allow development of a specific agent to reverse the process without the problems caused by current general bleaching agents.

Bleaching Agents

The two most commonly used bleaching agents are 30% to 35% hydrogen peroxide (Superoxol) and sodium perborate. They have been used with little alteration in technique for over 30 years.[3–5] Both are oxidizing agents, but Superoxol has about twice as much available oxygen as sodium perborate. This property makes it not only more reactive in bleaching, but also more likely to burn soft tissue. Close attention to protecting the patient's eyes and mucosa is necessary with both agents.

Although both bleaching agents are mildly caustic, their use causes few clinical problems. What is the concern in using these agents as long as the discoloration is reversed?

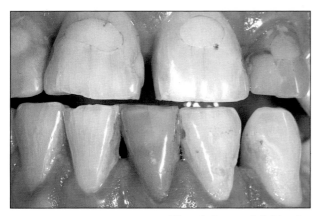 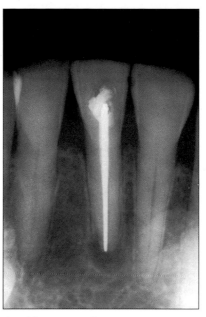

Figs 6-1a and 6-1b Coronal discoloration of a mandibular central incisor caused by cement and silver cone extending into the pulp chamber.

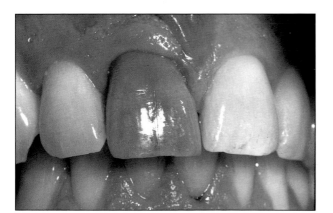

Trauma ⟶ Free RBC

Hemolysis ⟶ Hemoglobin

Iron + H_2S ⟶ Iron Sulfide

Figs 6-2a and 6-2b Discoloration has been attributed to necrotic pulp tissue and bacterial byproducts.[2]

Resorption

Figures 6-3a and 6-3b show a typical example of external cervical root resorption, which has been linked to intracoronal bleaching using hydrogen peroxide. Is this a rare example? The endodontic literature gives us an indication. Holmstrup et al bleached 69 teeth, evaluated them after three years, and found 0.0% incidence of resorption.[6] The same year, Friedman et al published a retrospective study of 58 teeth and found a resorption incidence of 6.9%.[7] In his study, one out of 12 teeth showed evidence of external cervical root resorption.

Was there something dissimilar in the design of these studies that accounts for the difference? Holmstrup and his colleagues used a walking bleach of sodium perborate and water. Friedman used 30% hydrogen peroxide and heat. At first glance, it appears the combination of Superoxol and heat is causing the problem. But is that the answer?

In order to address that question, it is helpful to review the original article by Harrington and Natkin associating intracoronal bleaching with external cervical root resorption.[8] Their patients had six characteristics in common:

1. All involved teeth became pulpless after a traumatic incident.
2. All patients were young, 11 to 15 years of age, at the time of trauma.
3. With one exception, the teeth were bleached 6 to 15 years after completion of the root canal therapy.
4. In all patients, Superoxol and heat were used during bleaching procedures.
5. In every patient, the resorption occurred in the cervical third of the root with no evidence of resorption elsewhere.
6. All patients denied further trauma after the initial traumatic incident.

Subsequent case reports began to discount some of these initial characteristics. Some teeth became pulpless due to an irreversible pulpitis caused by caries.[7,9,10] Others bleached immediately after endodontic therapy had external cervical root resorption.[8,14] Several were bleached using hydrogen peroxide without heat.[9,12,13] All case reports exhibited the characteristic resorption only at the CEJ, and no subsequent trauma was reported.

In all case reports of cervical root resorption, the teeth became pulpless before the patient had reached the age of 25. Furthermore, no barrier had been placed between the endodontic filling material and the pulp chamber.[7–15] Therefore, it appears that the age of the patient at the time the tooth became pulpless and the presence of a barrier may be as important as the type of bleaching agent and the use of heat during bleaching. This information leads to the rationale for the following bleaching technique.

> *It appears that the age of the patient at the time the tooth became pulpless and the presence of a barrier may be as important as the type of bleaching agent and the use of heat during bleaching.*

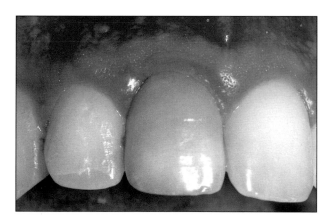
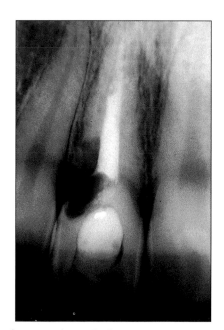

Figs 6-3a and 6-3b Example of external cervical root resorption. *(a)* Note the subtle pink color near the distogingival portion of the right central incisor. As shown by the periapical radiograph *(b)*, this hint of color often indicates hidden extensive tooth destruction.

Etiology

In 10% of all teeth, a defect can be found between the cementum and the enamel at the level of the cementoenamel junction (CEJ).[16] Therefore, dentinal tubules communicate between the root canal system and the periodontal membrane. If a tooth becomes pulpless when a patient is young, the dentinal tubules are relatively wide open, since sclerotic dentin can no longer form.

Dentinal tubules are oriented incisally (Fig 6-4a). Bleaching techniques recommend removal of gutta percha 1 to 3 mm apical to the labial CEJ, allowing the bleaching agent to diffuse incisally to lighten the cervical third of the crown.[17,19,25] The combination of bleach placed below the CEJ, a young pulpless tooth, and a potential defect at the junction of the cementum and enamel may allow the bleaching agent to diffuse through the patent dentinal tubules into the periodontal ligament below the epithelial attachment. This can initiate the inflammatory reaction that causes external root resorption at the cervical level.[8]

Barrier

The age of the patient at the time the tooth became pulpless and the lack of a bleach barrier appear to be critically important in the cause of external cervical root resorption. What can be done to control these factors?

Clinicians have no control over the age at which a tooth becomes pulpless, but they have control over the barrier. What is the perfect barrier? Where should it be located? What shape should it take? Which material is best?

Previous studies and techniques have suggested using the labial cementoenamel junction as a guide for barrier placement.[18,20] However, the CEJ is not level, but rather curves in an incisal direction on the proximal sides of the tooth (Fig 6-4b). A flat barrier leaves the proximal dentinal tubules unprotected; this critical area is the site where cervical resorption begins. The proximal tubules must be protected by the location and shape of the barrier.

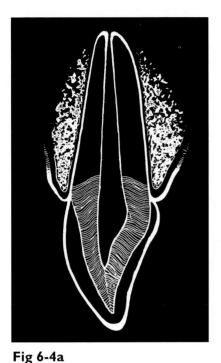

Fig 6-4a

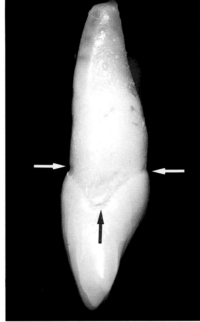

Fig 6-4b

Figs 6-4a and 6-4b Internal and external cervical anatomy. *(a)* Dentinal tubules are oriented incisally. *(b)* Note the proximal level of the CEJ curves in an incisal direction. A flat barrier, level with the labial CEJ, leaves a large triangle of unprotected dentinal tubules. The points of the triangle are identified by the three arrows. (Reprinted with permission from Steiner and West.[29])

Barrier Transfer

How is the location of the barrier determined? This step is essential to prevent resorption. Three periodontal probings are made with a custom "transfer periodontal probe." This is a periodontal probe carefully curved to match the labial contour of the tooth (Fig 6-5). First, a labial recording is made, followed by mesial and distal recordings (Figs 6-6a to 6-6f). These probings are made to determine the position of the epithelial attachment from the incisal edge of the tooth. The internal level of the barrier will be placed 1 mm incisal to the corresponding external probing of the epithelial attachment. This strategy blocks patent dentinal tubules that may communicate with the periodontal ligament apical to the epithelial attachment.

The idea is to block the dentinal tubules that lead from the pulp chamber apical to the epithelial attachment so that the internal bleaching agents stay within the access cavity. By subtracting 1 mm from each of the three probings, an internal template is created for the location and shape of the barrier. Positioning the palatal portion of the barrier equal or coronal to the barrier's proximal height protects the palatal CEJ without compromising the esthetic results. The resultant shape from a facial view is the "bobsled tunnel" outline (Fig 6-7a). This should be verified radiographically (Fig 6-7b). The outline form from the proximal resembles a "ski slope" (Fig 6-7c). A schematic drawing of the barrier is shown in Fig 6-7d.

There is also an esthetic reason for avoiding the CEJ as a guide for barrier placement. In an instance of gingival recession, the root would not be completely bleached using the CEJ guideline as a reference (Figs 6-8a and 6-8b). Instead, a more biologically critical and esthetically essential landmark is to relate the barrier to the epithelial attachment.

After identification and transfer of the level of the epithelial attachment, the barrier may be placed. In preliminary studies, intermediate restorative material (IRM, L.D. Caulk), zinc oxyphosphate, and dentin sealants failed to provide adequate bleach barriers. However, carefully placed Cavit (ESPE/Premier) or light-cured glass-ionomer cements may offer promise as barrier materials. Research to identify the best barrier material is ongoing.[19–22]

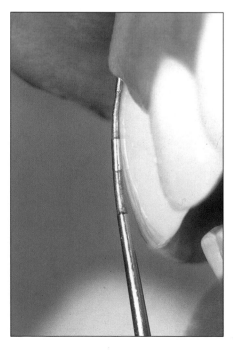

Fig 6-5 Transfer periodontal probe. A curved periodontal probe facilitates accurate measurement of the epithelial attachment from the incisal edge.

Figs 6-6a to 6-6f Barrier transfer. The external level of the epithelial attachment is recorded at the labial, mesial, and distal *(a, c, and e, respectively)*. The internal level of the barrier is placed 1 mm incisal to the corresponding external probing *(b, d, and f)*. (Reprinted with permission from Steiner and West.[29])

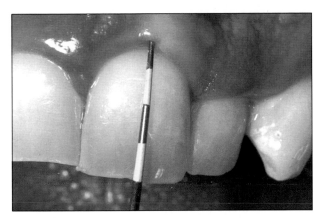

Fig 6-6a

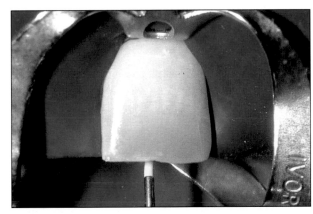

Fig 6-6b

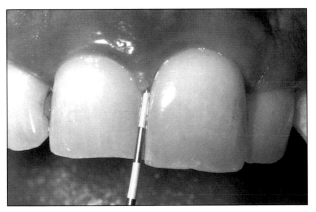

Fig 6-6c

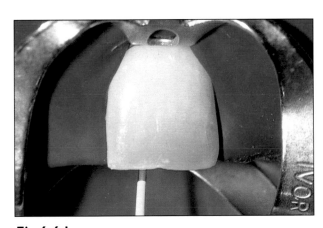

Fig 6-6d

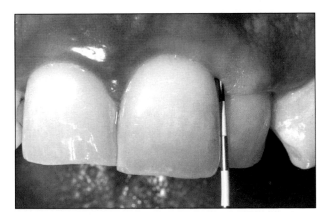

Fig 6-6e

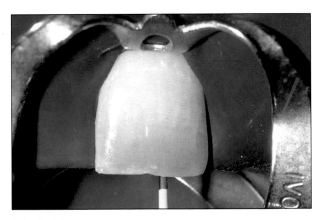

Fig 6-6f

Figs 6-7a to 6-7d Barrier outline forms.

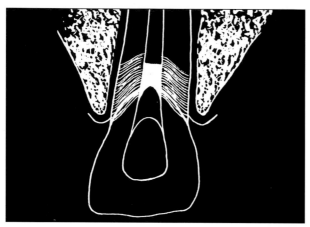

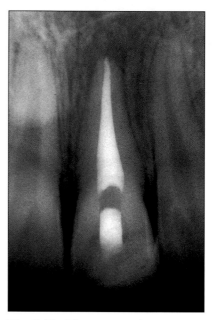

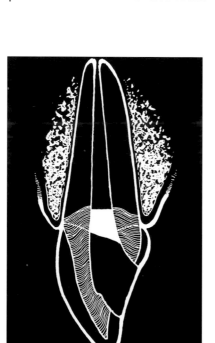

Fig 6-7a The facial outline of a barrier appears as a "bobsled tunnel." (Figs 6-7a to 6-7d reprinted with permission from Steiner and West.[29])

Fig 6-7b The correct barrier shape is verified by a radiograph.

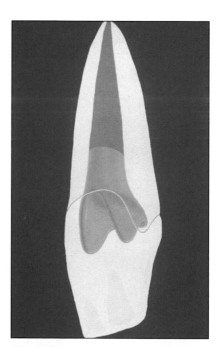

Fig 6-7c The proximal shape of a barrier is a "ski slope."

Fig 6-7d Schematic of an ideal barrier. The contours of the internal barrier "wings" conform to the external proximal epithelial attachment to protect the dentinal tubules.

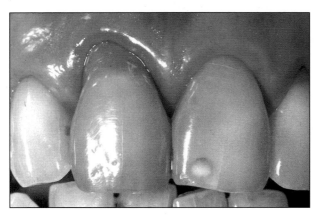

Fig 6-8a Using the CEJ as a guide for barrier placement prevents the root from being bleached in instances of gingival recession.

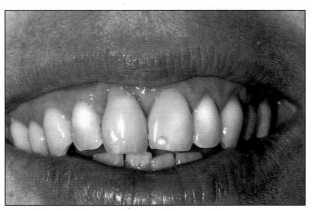

Fig 6-8b An unbleached root creates an unesthetic result in a patient with a high lip line.

Recipe

This section focuses not on external bleaching of teeth with vital pulps, but rather on internal bleaching of pulpless teeth. What are the guidelines for a safe and successful bleach? Which teeth are ideal case selections? Which technique is best? What are the problems and solutions of nonvital bleaching?

Case Selection

Which teeth are amenable to intracoronal bleaching? Successful bleaching depends upon two important criteria. First, the root-canal obturation must be complete. In order to prevent an endodontic failure, the root canal system must be filled in three dimensions. Second, the remaining tooth structure must be intact.[1] The ideal tooth for nonvital bleaching is a discolored tooth with an unrestored crown (Figs 6-9a and 6-9b). If minor restorations are necessary, the tooth should be bleached first. Then the color of the restorative material may be matched to the resulting tooth color. If the tooth requires significant restoration, it should be restored with a porcelain laminate or full crown (Figs 6-9c and 6-9d). When staining is caused by alloy restorations or endodontic sealers containing silver, the bleaching effect is less predictable. These teeth may also be better candidates for crowns or laminates.

Figs 6-9a to 6-9d Proper case selection.

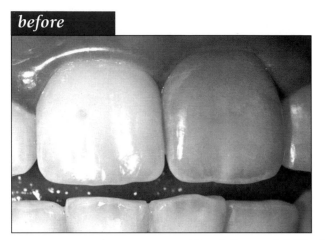

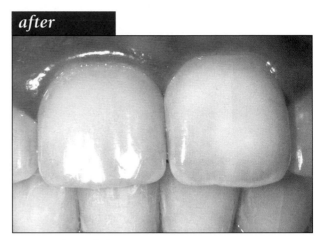

Figs 6-9a and 6-9b An unrestored tooth is ideal for nonvital bleaching.

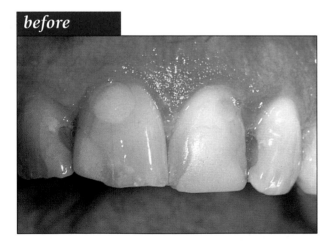

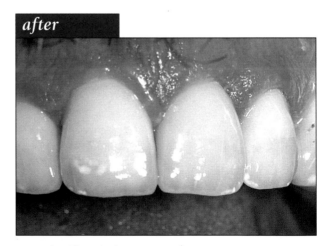

Figs 6-9c and 6-9d Place a crown if a tooth has significant restorations. (Restorative treatment: Dr Frank Spear)

Treatment Technique

Diagnose

Evaluate the vitality of the pulp with thermal and electric pulp testing (Fig 6-10). If a radiographic lesion of endodontic origin is present, an access cavity without anesthesia may be used to confirm the diagnosis of a pulpless tooth. Where previous endodontic treatment exists, confirm the adequacy of the obturation and the health of the surrounding bone (Fig 6-11).

Record shade

A photograph and a shade guide provide legal and treatment references to measure the progress of color enhancement.

Record barrier probings

These periodontal measurements will be used to establish the location and shape of the barrier between the root canal filling material and the pulp chamber.

Isolate the tooth

A thorough dental prophylaxis of the pulpless tooth as well as adjacent teeth will reveal the true color of the tooth. Adapt a well-fitted rubber dam to isolate only the tooth to be bleached or the two adjacent teeth as well. Three-tooth isolation is useful for a comparison of adjacent shades (Fig 6-12a). Cervical ligation with dental floss will protect gingival tissues by maximizing the seal and will allow better visibility of the enamel. This permits accurate observation of the critical cervical region during the bleaching process. Be sure to protect the patient and treatment team with eyewear, gloves, and masks (Fig 6-12b).

Prepare the access cavity

The design of the access cavity should follow normal endodontic access guidelines. After canal obturation, the access cavity must be meticulously cleaned by removing any remaining necrotic debris, root canal filling material, or endodontic sealers.

Transfer barrier probings

Transfer the external periodontal probings into the pulp chamber to create an outline for the internal barrier.

Place barrier material (Figs 6-13a to 6-13c)

If glass ionomer is used, place cement onto a straight lentulo spiral mounted in a latch-type slow-speed handpiece. Using a rubber stop to identify the labial depth of the barrier, spin the glass-ionomer cement into the access cavity to this predetermined level. It is important to carry the barrier material to the gutta-percha base and then activate the handpiece so that the barrier material will flow flat. This technique will also eliminate voids between the barrier and the gutta percha. As the glass-ionomer cement becomes viscous, use the barrier probe to drag the cement up the proximal walls of the access cavity, thereby completing and confirming the level of the internal protective barrier. Glass ionomer is light-cured first from the labial and then from the lingual access cavity.

If a cement such as Cavit is used to form the barrier, place a small cone of Cavit on the end of a plugger and pack it against the gutta percha. Then use the back of a spoon excavator to slope the cement from 1 mm coronal to the labial epithelial attachment toward the lingual external margin of the access cavity. Press the cement against the proximal walls to the proper level. Use a wet cotton pellet to accelerate the set of the cement.

Introduce bleaching solution

Either place a cotton pellet saturated with Superoxol against the labial wall or syringe fresh 35% hydrogen peroxide into the pulp chamber to a level just inside the cavosurface of the access cavity.

Thermocatalytically activate bleach

Activate the bleaching agent with an appropriate heat bleaching instrument as the Analytic Technology 5003 Touch 'n' Heat (Analytic Technology) (Fig 6-14a). Place the bleaching wand into the solution and activate the probe with a setting of 2 to 3 (Fig 6-14b). Heat the solution for 2 minutes, then change the Superoxol. Repeat this procedure once. At this point, external brushes saturated with bleach may be used on the facial surface to enhance the bleaching effect (Fig 6-14c). Caldwell claimed that heating the bleach solution will increase the bleaching rate of 35% hydrogen peroxide about 200 times.[23]

Do not use a heated endodontic plugger with the free liquid bleach in the chamber. The uncontrolled temperature of the instrument causes the solution to boil out of the access. When using a heated plugger, place a bleach-saturated cotton pellet against the labial wall. Activate the bleaching agent by repeatedly placing the instrument against the saturated cotton pellet until the bleach has evaporated. Repeat this process up to three times.

Rinse and close

Some of the color change during heat bleaching may be due to dehydration of the tooth. Place a temporary and evaluate the tooth after rehydration. If, at the end of heat bleaching, the shade still remains darker than the adjacent teeth, rinse the chamber and place a walking bleach. Evaluate in 3 to 7 days and repeat as necessary.

Place walking bleach

The walking bleach procedure (Fig 6-15a) is effective, efficient, and has the advantage of evaluating color over time. It allows patients to see their teeth in different light during their daily activities.

Place a thick mix of sodium perborate and Superoxol, or sodium perborate and water. The mixtures are dried by blotting to produce a stiff paste (Fig 6-15b). This facilitates placement of the material. It can be carried to the access cavity with an amalgam carrier and pressed into place with a large amalgam condenser or endodontic plugger (Fig 6-15c). If the paste is wiped into place with a plastic instrument, some material will inevitably be scraped onto the access cavosurface. Use a damp cotton pellet to remove the excess. The cavosurface must be clean to permit an adequate seal and prevent leakage of the bleach material between appointments (Fig 6-15d).

Insert temporary seal

After placing the walking bleach into the chamber, a 2-mm layer of Cavit can be used as a fast, easy, and effective temporary (Fig 6-16). Wipe the first layer against the entire inner cavosurface rim. Spread another layer of Cavit gently into the remaining space. Wipe the excess toward the cavosurface with alcohol on a cotton pellet.

Determine duration of walking bleach

Leave the walking bleach mixture in place for 2 to 7 days, or until the patient notices that the tooth is as light or slightly lighter than the adjacent teeth.

Combination bleaching

Thermocatalytic and walking bleaches may be used separately or in combination. Which bleaching method is best? The effectiveness and rate of the bleaching change appears inversely proportional to the safety of the method. A walking bleach of sodium perborate and water bleaches teeth between 50% and 60% of the time, but no case reports of resorption have been associated with its use.[6,25,27]

The combination of Superoxol and heat followed by a walking bleach using a mixture of Superoxol and sodium perborate is effective in bleaching teeth about 90% of the time.[25] The impression is that an increased chance of resorption is possible with this combination. However, if used with an adequate barrier and in a tooth that became pulpless after the patient was older than 25 years, the chance of problems appears minimal.

Step 15

Restore access

When the color has been lightened sufficiently, isolate the tooth with a rubber dam and clean the access cavity carefully to remove all traces of temporary material. Acid-etch the enamel cavosurface, wash, and dry (Fig 6-17a). Place a layered light-activated composite resin (Fig 6-17b). Light-cure from the labial surface and then the lingual surface (Figs 6-17c and 6-17d). This sequence may cause the composite to shrink toward the axial walls and reduce microleakage.[26] Fill the remaining chamber with light-cured composite in the same labiolingual sequence. Finish using appropriate polishing procedures for maximum esthetic results (Figs 6-18a to 6-18d).

Although acid-etching the cavosurface and filling the chamber with a light-cured composite appears to reduce the rate of rediscoloration, microleakage remains a problem.[28] The extent to which it can be eliminated will determine the permanence of the bleaching effect.

Figs 6-10 and 6-11 Diagnosis.

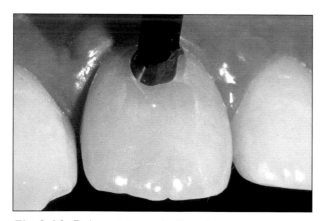

Fig 6-10 Determining pulpal vitality.

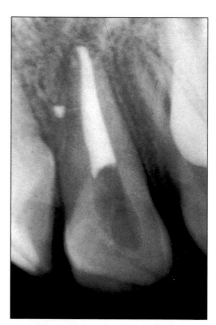

Fig 6-11 Oblique radiograph of maxillary central incisor showing the root canal system filled in three dimensions and healthy surrounding bone.

Figs 6-12a and 6-12b Bleaching protection.

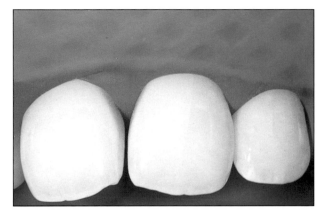

Fig 6-12a Gingival tissue is protected by a well-fitting rubber dam.

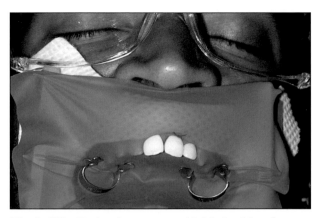

Fig 6-12b Patient's eyes are shielded with safety glasses.

Figs 6-13a to 6-13c Barrier placement.

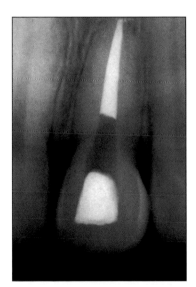

Fig 6-13a Three-dimensional endodontic filling prior to barrier placement. The gutta percha ends about 2 mm apical to the CEJ.

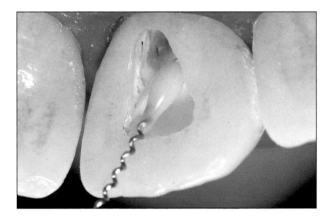

Fig 6-13b Glass ionomer is carried into the canal with a lentulo spiral.

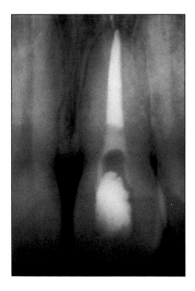

Fig 6-13c Radiograph of barrier showing "bobsled tunnel" shape.

Figs 6-14a to 6-14c Thermocatalytic technique.

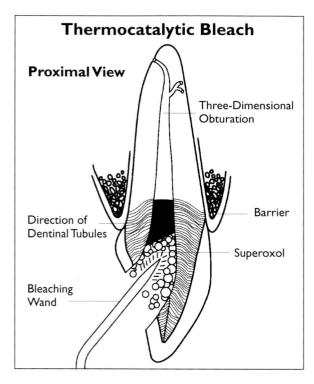

Fig 6-14a Placement of Superoxol and heating unit. (Reprinted with permission from Cohen S, Burns R [eds]. Pathways of the Pulp, ed 6. St Louis: Mosby, 1994.)

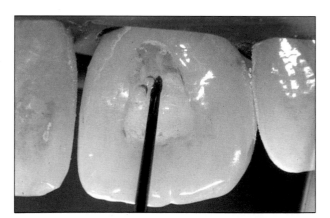

Fig 6-14b Effect of Superoxol is accelerated internally by heat bleaching instrument.

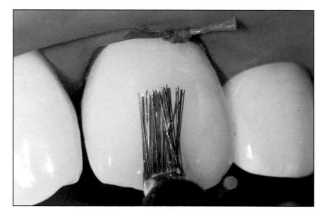

Fig 6-14c Heated external brushes carry Superoxol to the buccal surface to enhance bleaching effect.

Figs 6-15a to 6-15d Walking bleach. _____

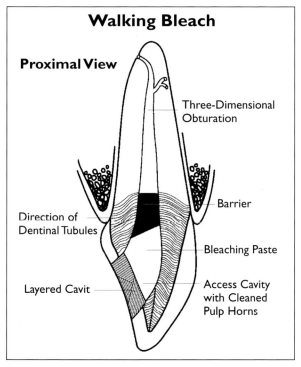

Walking Bleach

Proximal View

Three-Dimensional Obturation

Barrier

Direction of Dentinal Tubules

Bleaching Paste

Layered Cavit

Access Cavity with Cleaned Pulp Horns

Fig 6-15a Placement of bleaching paste and Cavit. (Reprinted with permission from Cohen S, Burns R [eds]. Pathways of the Pulp, ed 6. St Louis: Mosby, 1994.)

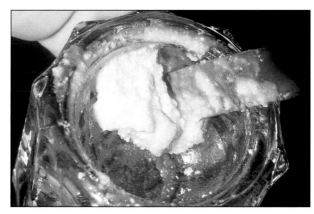

Fig 6-15b Walking bleach of sodium perborate and water mixed to a thick paste.

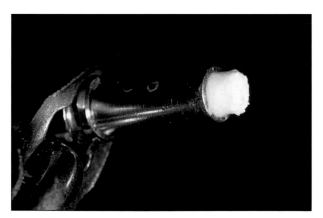

Fig 6-15c Paste is carried to the pulp chamber with an amalgam carrier.

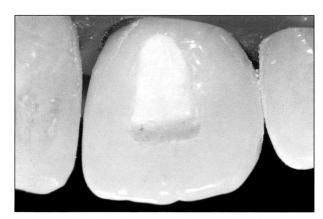

Fig 6-15d Two millimeters of space should be left for Cavit temporary.

Fig 6-16 Temporary seal.

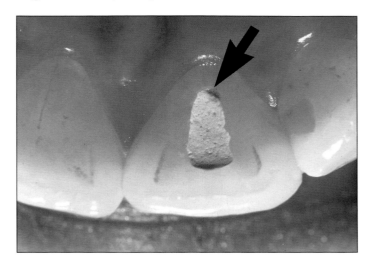

Fig 6-16 Oxygen released from the bleaching agents may rupture a thin temporary seal, eliminating the bleaching effect *(arrow)*.

Figs 6-17a to 6-17d Access restoration.

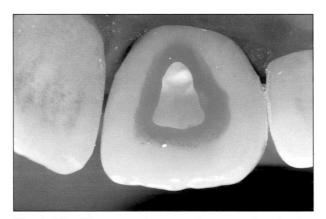

Fig 6-17a The enamel cavosurface is acid-etched.

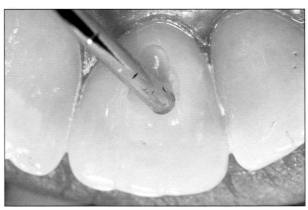

Fig 6-17b Light-cured composite resin is placed in layers.

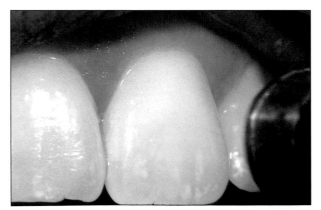

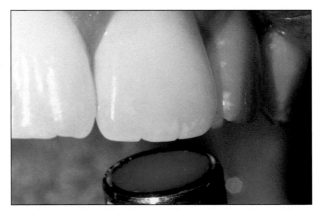

Figs 6-17c and 6-17d The composite resin should be light-cured from the labial surface first, then from the lingual surface. This sequence may reduce microleakage.

Figs 6-18a to 6-18d Nonvital bleaching is a conservative technique to renew an esthetic smile.

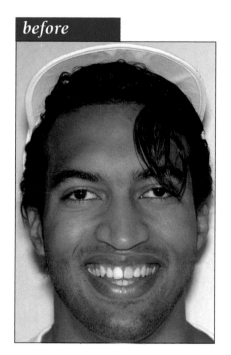

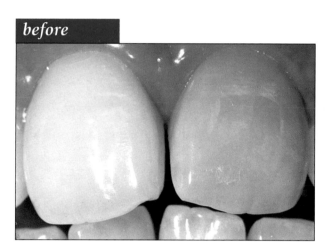

Figs 6-18a and 6-18b Discolored maxillary left central incisor.

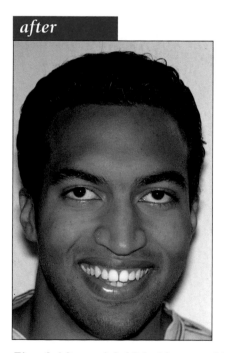

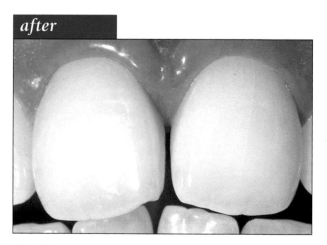

Figs 6-18c and 6-18d After combination bleaching.

Recommendations for Safe Bleaching

1. Excellent Endodontic Treatment
Excellent endodontic treatment is required to prevent leaking of the bleaching agent through underfilled foramina.

2. Patient History
All published case reports of external cervical root resorption have occurred in patients whose teeth became pulpless before age 25. Patent dentinal tubules appear to be a factor in allowing bleach to diffuse more readily into the periodontal membrane space. No report of cervical root resorption after bleaching with sodium perborate and water has been published. It may be prudent to use this combination when bleaching pulpless teeth in young patients or in teeth that became pulpless before age 25.

3. Barrier
The location, shape, and materials of a protective barrier have been discussed. Its presence appears critical in preventing resorption.

4. No Etch
Evaluators were unable to distinguish a significant difference between the results of walking bleach procedures carried out with dentinal etching of the pulp chambers and those bleached without etching.[24] Since etching opens the dentinal tubules, having an adequate barrier becomes more important. Should the barrier fail, etching may increase the potential of external cervical root resorption.

5. New Superoxol and Sodium Perborate
Bleaching agents lose their effectiveness over time. Superoxol may lose about 50% of its oxidizing strength in a 6-month period.[25]

6. Recalls
Resorption has been detected as early as 6 months after intracoronal bleaching.[10] Most cervical root resorption has been detected after 2 years and was often too advanced to salvage the tooth. Early detection improves the possibility of arresting and repairing the problem.

Basic Safety Guidelines

Safest Bleach

1. Tooth became pulpless in a patient over 25 years of age.
2. Properly positioned barrier.
3. Sodium perborate plus water.

Least Safe Bleach

1. Tooth became pulpless in a patient under 25 years of age.
2. No barrier, or incorrectly placed barrier.
3. Superoxol plus heat.

Troubleshooting in Nonvital Bleaching

Three different bleaching approaches—thermocatalytic, walking, and combination—may be used to bleach pulpless teeth. Recommendations for the proper and safe use of these treatments have been discussed in this chapter. The table on pages 124 and 125 and Figs 6-19 to 6-27 present cases in which these approaches were used to meet bleaching challenges. By following the recommendations outlined for case selection and treatment technique, and by integrating endodontic and esthetic restorative principles, predictable and safe bleaching of pulpless teeth can be mastered.

Troubleshooting in Nonvital Bleaching

Problem	Possible Causes	Solution
1. Color does not improve with bleaching (Figs 6-19a to 6-19c).	• Old Superoxol. • Insufficient bleaching time. • Discoloration requires combination bleaching. • Defective temporary seal.	• Obtain fresh Superoxol. • Perform additional walking bleaches and/or combination bleaching with heat.
2. Staining from metal- or silver-containing sealers (Figs 6-20a to 6-21c).	• Silver cone extended into chamber. • Amalgam placed in access cavity.	• Remove silver cone or amalgam. Retreat with gutta percha and sealer. • Perform nonvital bleaching with barrier in place.
3. Patient tastes walking bleach mixture.	• Defective seal. • Too much sodium perborate used. • Walking bleach mix too thin.	• Flush all walking bleach mix from tooth and seal properly. • Be sure there is clean, dry tooth structure between the packed sodium perborate and the cavosurface of the access cavity.
4. Discolored tooth is next to implant (Figs 6-22a to 6-22c).	• Dictated by treatment plan.	• Perform nonvital bleaching with an adequate barrier for safety.
5. Gingival third fails to bleach.	• Gingival third dentin thicker. • Barrier covers gingival third, preventing bleaching of this area.	• Rebleach gingival third only. • Remove excess labial barrier while staying 1 mm incisal to labial epithelial attachment (see Figs 6-7a to 6-7d).
6. Patient reports stinging during bleaching.	• Leakage of bleaching material onto tissue.	• Remove rubber dam and flush area thoroughly. • Use smaller rubber dam holes and tuck rubber dam using explorer and air. • Use protective gingival seals or Vaseline over gingiva before rubber dam. • Improve ligation and confine bleaching materials to the chamber.

Troubleshooting in Nonvital Bleaching *(continued)*

Problem	Possible Causes	Solution
7. Discolored tooth has endodontic post (Figs 6-23a to 6-23f).	• Inappropriate use of post where intact crown is present.	• Remove post and retreat with gutta percha and sealer. • Use a nonvital bleaching technique to restore esthetic match.
8. Color relapse (Figs 6-24a to 6-24c).	• Microleakage in the access cavity.	• Remove lingual access material, rebleach, and repair access with acid-etched, layered, light-cured restorative materials. • Be aware of new techniques to reduce microleakage.
9. Tooth shade is too light after bleaching.	• Walking bleach left in too long. • Failure to compare color change during thermo-catalytic bleaching.	• Consider access restorative materials that will darken the tooth. • Best solution is prevention and better monitoring of bleaching process.
10. Tooth is discolored due to calcified chamber. (Figs 6-25a to 6-27a).	• Increased dentin thickness changes natural appearance of tooth.	• Perform endodontic treatment followed by nonvital bleaching (Figs 6-25a to 6-25d). • Make normal access cavity. Place base and perform nonvital bleaching without endodontic treatment (Fig 6-26a to 6-26d). • External bleaching with Superoxol and external heating instrument and/or dual-activated bleaching paste (Figs 6-27a to 6-27c).

Figs 6-19a to 6-22c Troubleshooting in nonvital bleaching: different techniques. ———————

before

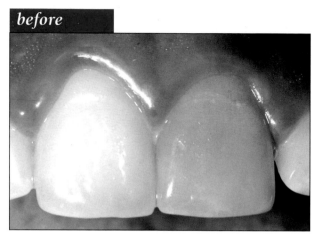

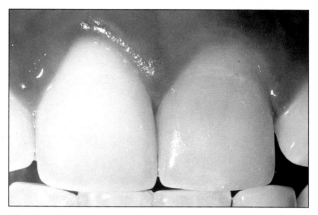

Fig 6-19a Maxillary left central incisor before bleaching.

Fig 6-19b After one walking bleach, color only partially improves.

after

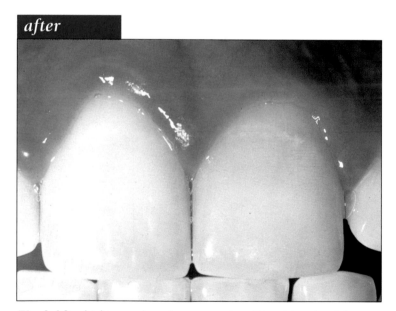

Fig 6-19c Lighter color after second walking bleach with new Superoxol (Union Broach).

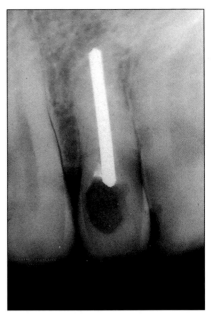

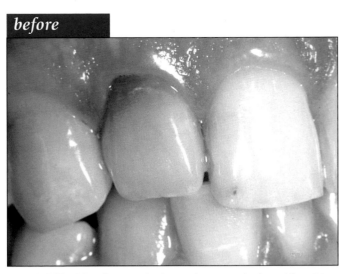

Fig 6-20b Maxillary right lateral incisor before bleaching.

Fig 6-20a Silver cone staining of maxillary right lateral incisor. Radiograph is before retreatment with gutta percha and sealer.

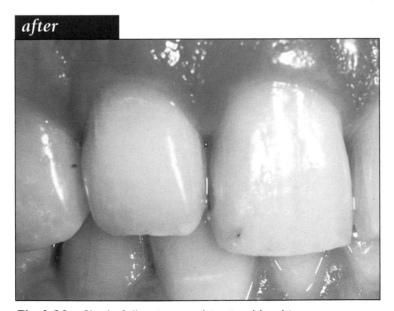

Fig 6-20c Shade following combination bleaching.

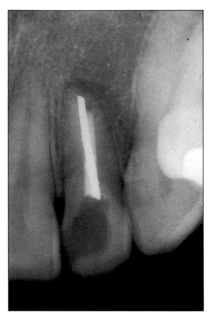

Fig 6-21a Radiograph of maxillary left lateral incisor before retreatment with gutta percha and sealer.

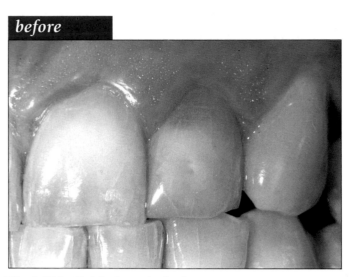

Fig 6-21b Original tooth shade.

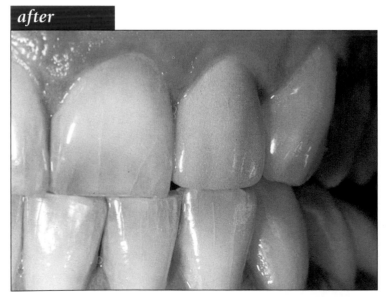

Fig 6-21c Porcelain-fused-to-metal crown is an alternative solution. This example demonstrates the difficulty of a perfect restorative match.

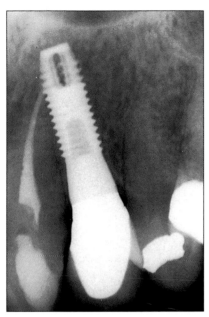

Fig 6-22a Radiograph of maxillary left lateral incisor next to single-tooth implant.

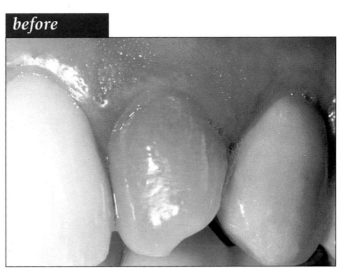

Fig 6-22b Before nonvital bleaching.

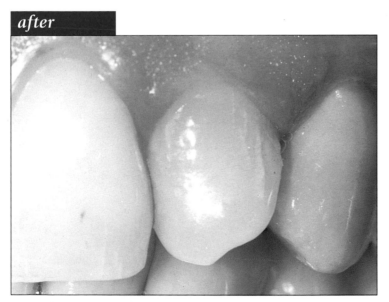

Fig 6-22c Bleached tooth resembling color of adjacent natural tooth and implant-supported restoration.

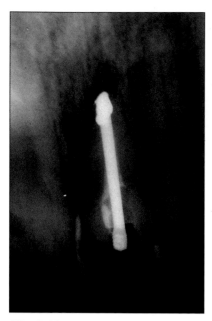

Fig 6-23a Periapical radiograph of maxillary left central incisor with post extending into chamber.

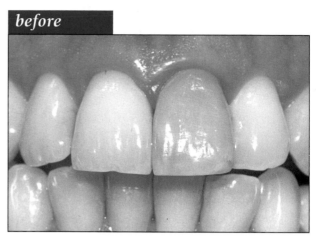

Fig 6-23b Clinical appearance of discolored incisor.

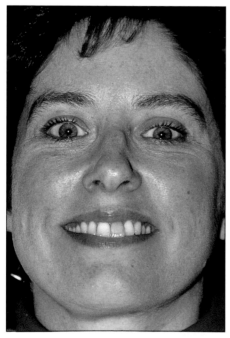

Fig 6-23c Patient before post removal, retreatment, and nonvital bleaching sequence.

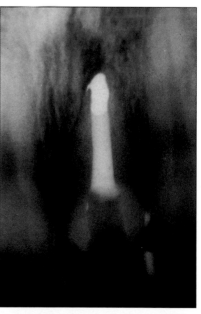

Fig 6-23d Radiograph of post removed and endodontic retreatment with gutta percha and sealer prior to barrier placement.

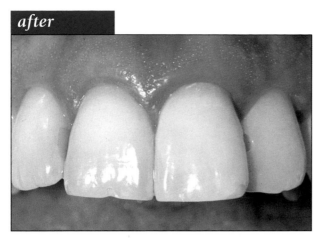

after

Fig 6-23e Favorable color alteration after nonvital bleaching.

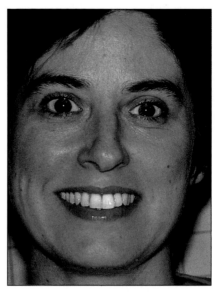

Fig 6-23f Successful result enhances smile.

Figs 6-24a to 6-24c Troubleshooting in nonvital bleaching: color relapse. _____

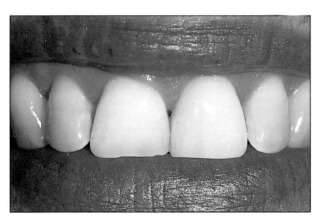

Fig 6-24a Maxillary left central incisor (different patient) immediately after nonvital bleaching.

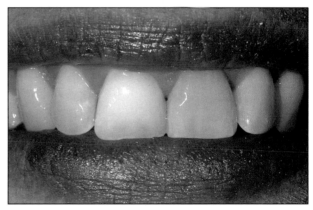

Fig 6-24b Three-year color relapse. Access cavity was restored with self-curing composite resin and no etching.

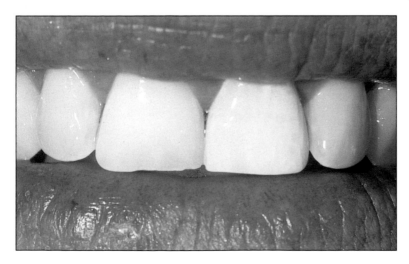

Fig 6-24c Successful rebleaching using a walking bleach. Special attention is given to etching the access cavosurface of the chamber and restoring it with layered light-cured composite resin in order to minimize coronal microleakage.

Figs 6-25a to 6-27c Troubleshooting in nonvital bleaching: calcified pulp chamber.

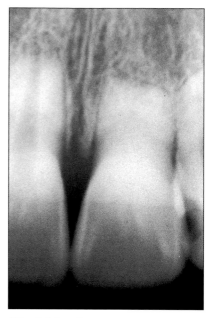

Fig 6-25a Pretreatment radiograph of calcified vital maxillary central incisor.

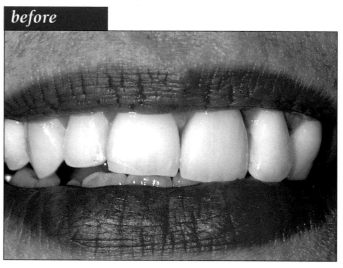

Fig 6-25b Pretreatment photograph of typical darkening due to calcification.

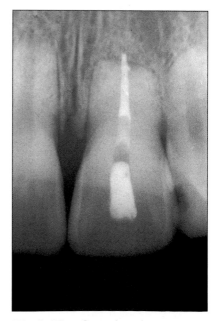

Fig 6-25c Completed conventional endodontic treatment.

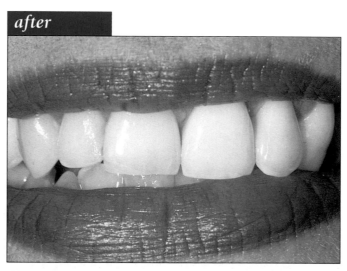

Fig 6-25d After intracoronal walking bleach.

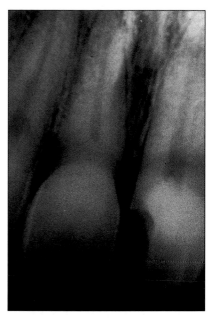

Fig 6-26a Pretreatment radiograph of vital maxillary right central incisor.

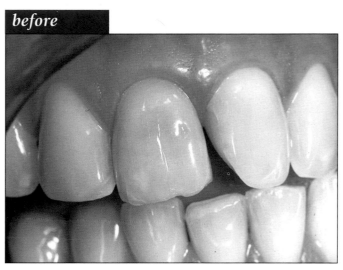

Fig 6-26b Discoloration due to calcified pulp chamber.

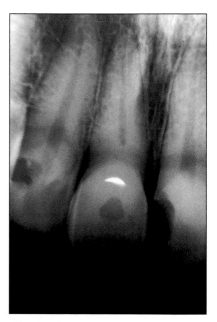

Fig 6-26c Radiograph of completed access cavity only with a ZOE base.

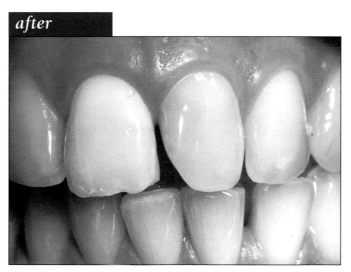

Fig 6-26d Final successful result prior to restoration of adjacent maxillary left central incisor. Patients must be cautioned there is a risk of pulpal necrosis with this approach, and that conventional or surgical treatment may become necessary.

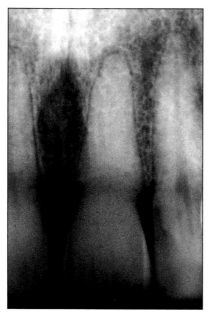

Fig 6-27a Radiograph of discolored vital maxillary left central incisor with severe calcific degeneration of root canal system.

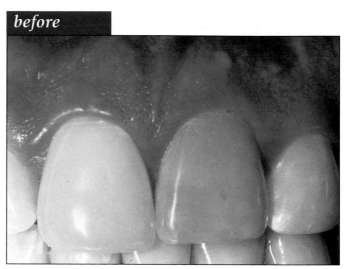

Fig 6-27b Discoloration due to obliteration of canal space by sclerotic dentin.

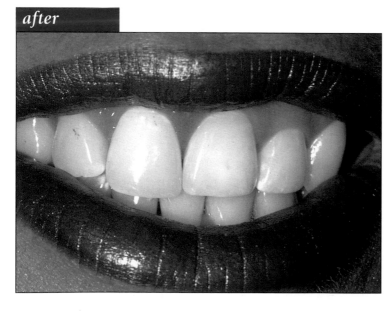

Fig 6-27c Favorable esthetic result using external heat bleaching with brushes and hydrogen peroxide. This procedure often requires a considerable increase in chairtime and appointments. Other methods include single-tooth home vital bleaching and external dual-activated bleaching.

References

1. Goldstein RE, Feinman RA. Bleaching of vital and non-vital teeth. In: Cohen S, Burns R (eds). Pathways of the Pulp, ed 5. St Louis: Mosby, 1991: 628–639.

2. Grossman LI. Endodontic Practice, ed 5. Philadelphia: Lea and Febiger, 1960: 385.

3. Pearson HH. Bleaching of the discolored pulpless tooth. J Am Dent Assoc 1958;56:64–68.

4. Nutting EB, Poe GS. A new combination for bleaching teeth. J South Calif St Dent Assoc 1963;31:289–291.

5. Spasser HF. A simple bleaching technique using sodium perborate. NY St Dent J 1961;27:332–334.

6. Holmstrup G, Palm AM, Lambjerg-Hansen H. Bleaching of discolored root-filled teeth. Endodont Dent Traumatol 1988;4:197–201.

7. Friedman S, Rotstein I, Libfeld H, Stabholz A, and Helmig II. Incidence of external root resorption and esthetic results in 58 bleached pulpless teeth. Endodont Dent Traumatol 1988;4:23–26.

8. Harrington GW, Natkin E. External resorption associated with bleaching of pulpless teeth. J Endodont 1979;5:344–348.

9. Lado EA, Stanley HR, Weisman MI. Cervical resorption in bleached teeth. Oral Surg 1983;55:78–80.

10. Cvek M, Lindvall AM. External root resorption following bleaching of pulpless teeth with oxygen peroxide. Endodont Dent Traumatol 1985;1:56–60.

11. Latcham NL. Management of a patient with postbleaching cervical resorption. A clinical report. J Prosthet Dent 1991;65: 603–605.

12. Latcham NL. Postbleaching cervical resorption. J Endodont 1986; 12:262–265.

13. Goon W, Cohen S, Borer R. External cervical root resorption following bleaching. J Endodont 1986;12:414–418.

14. Gimlin DR, Schindler WG. The management of postbleaching cervical resorption. J Endodont 1990;16:292–297.

15. Montgomery S. External cervical resorption after bleaching a pulpless tooth. Oral Surg 1984;57:203–206.

16. Ten Cate AR. Oral Histology: Development, Structure, and Function, ed 2. St Louis: Mosby, 1985:234.

17. Arens D. The role of bleaching in esthetics. Dent Clin North Am 1989;33:319–336.

18. Warren W, Wong M, Ingram T. An in vitro comparison of bleaching agents on the crowns and roots of discolored teeth. J Endodont 1990;16:463–467.

19. Costas FL, Wong M. Intracoronal isolating barriers: Effect of location on root leakage and effectiveness of bleaching agents. J Endodont 1991;17:365–368.

20. Rotstein I, Zyskind D, Lewinstein I, Baumberger N. Effect of different protective base materials on hydrogen peroxide leakage during intracoronal bleaching in vitro. J Endodont 1992;18:114–117.

21. McInerney ST, Zillich R. Evaluation of internal sealing ability of three materials. J Endodont 1992;18:376–378.

22. Smith JJ, Cunningham CJ, Montgomery S. Cervical canal leakage after internal bleaching procedures. J Endodont 1992;18:476–481.

23. Caldwell CB. Bleaching vital or nonvital teeth. J Calif Dent Assoc 1966;42:234–235.

24. Casey LJ, Schindler WG, Murata SM, Burgess JO. The use of dentinal etching with endodontic bleaching procedures. J Endodont 1989;15:535–538.

25. Ho S, Goerig AC. An in vitro comparison of different bleaching agents in the discolored tooth J Endodont 1989;15:106–111.

26. Lemon R. Bleaching and restoring endodontically treated teeth. Curr Opin Dent 1991;1:754–759.

27. Rotstein I, Alkind M, Mor C, Tarabeah A, Friedman S. In vitro efficacy of sodium perborate preparations used for intracoronal bleaching of discolored non-vital teeth. Endodont Dent Traumatol 1991:7:177–180.

28. Wilcox LR, Diaz-Arnold A. Coronal microleakage of permanent lingual access restorations in endodontically treated anterior teeth. J Endodont 1989;15:584–587.

29. Steiner DR, West JD. A method to determine the location and shape of an intracoronal bleach barrier. J Endodont 1994;20:304–306.

Total Team Care in Combination Bleaching

When bleaching is a part of a broader treatment plan for the overall improvement of a smile, teamwork between the dental professionals involved is essential.

As dental treatments for esthetic needs become more common, health-care professionals must become more responsible for being knowledgeable about each others' specialties. It is important that each specialist fully comprehend what is currently available within the interdisciplinary realm for their patients' total esthetic care and smile enhancement. Dental disciplines from general dentistry to orthodontics, periodontics, oral surgery, orthognathic surgery, plastic and reconstructive surgery, and other specialties should understand the role of bleaching and similar esthetic restorative modalities in creating the desired look in each case.

By the same token, the general dentist must recognize that patients frequently will come to him or her for advice on how to achieve a more attractive smile before they consult specialists for other needs. The generalist is often the best person both to develop an integrated comprehensive treatment plan and to assemble and coordinate the patient's entire dental team. Be sure to document all advice regarding the treatment plan and post-treatment

> *The generalist is often the best person both to develop an integrated comprehensive treatment plan and to assemble and coordinate the patient's entire dental team.*

recommendations. This documentation should be in the form of letters to *both* the patient and the specialists to whom you refer the patient. Since treatment plans vary according to each patient's needs, you must inform your referral specialists of the long-term plans for the patient after he or she completes the individual specialty treatments. For example, if you believe your patient's teeth will need cosmetic contouring following orthodontic treatment, specify whether you, the orthodontist, or yet some other specialist on the team you have assembled will be performing the contouring. Definitive treatment-plan documentation is particularly necessary for bleaching, since so many dental disciplines now offer bleaching, especially matrix bleaching, as part of their services.

In our own practice, which is concerned predominantly with esthetic dentistry, fully half our patients receive orthodontic consultation; a somewhat smaller proportion consult with an orthognathic surgeon as well. Consultation involving the entire team and all treatment options is essential to a good dentist-patient relationship. A dentist should never hear from a patient that he or she did not provide the patient with all the various options available for esthetic improvement or functional health prior to, following, or even during specialty treatment.

Every treatment plan involving bleaching in combination with other dental procedures will be different, and it is this teamwork that will determine each patient's specific plan and ultimate success. Earlier chapters have described how to select patients who are appropriate for bleaching and to eliminate those for whom it is contraindicated. Once the decision is made that bleaching is a viable modality, the following guidelines can serve as a blueprint for creating the team that can provide that patient the complete spectrum of needed care.

> *No plan for esthetic treatment should be made final until all necessary specialists have been consulted.*

Bleaching in Conjunction with Restorative Dental Care

Defective Restorations

Any defective restorations in the tooth must be repaired before bleaching because of the possibility of penetration of the bleaching solution. Repairs may consist of merely etching and resealing the margins as a temporary measure or actually replacing the restoration with a lighter shade. If patients with old restorations request bleaching, it must be explained to them before treatment that the teeth lighten, but restorations do not and would need to be replaced to match the color change. Patients should be fully informed that this matching process is not simple (Figs 7-1a to 7-1c). If the placed restoration is a lighter color than the teeth, it is always possible to rebleach the labial surface of the teeth to develop a closer blend.

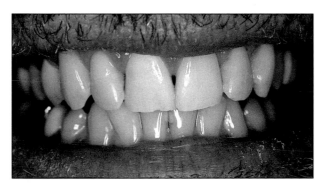

Fig 7-1a Leaking or defective restorations should either be replaced or etched and sealed for protection prior to the first bleaching.

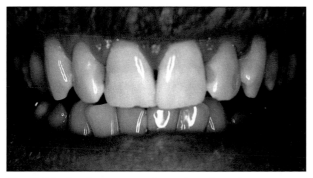

Fig 7-1b Replacement of any discolored restorations with a lighter shade of composite resin should not occur until 2 to 3 weeks following the last bleaching treatment.

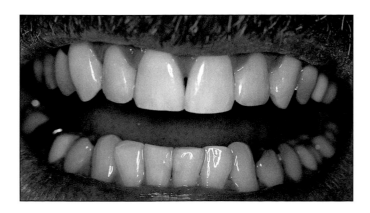

Fig 7-1c Waiting a short time following the last bleaching treatment assures the best possible color match with class 3 composites.

Direct Composite Bonding

Many patients are undecided whether to attempt color change with direct composite resin, porcelain veneers, or bleaching. Because your treatment planning is based on the utilization of a full spectrum of options, you can reassure the patient that in an integrated approach any lightening initially produced by bleaching can be useful in facilitating the use of lighter restorations with decreased amounts of opacifier within the composite or laminate veneer, thus allowing for a more natural translucent appearance. This is possible because the color of the bleached teeth bleed through the new, partially transparent restorations.

For teeth with a variegated pattern of stains, it may be possible to bleach the teeth entirely and then bond the entire labial surfaces of teeth or just those regions that do not respond well (Figs 7-2a to 7-2c).

Before deciding whether to veneer or bleach, carefully examine the patient's enamel, tooth position, and arch form.

When teeth have definitive white or brown stains, it may be preferable to use a combination of microabrasion and bleaching prior to bonding in order to diminish these discolorations when bleaching alone does not accomplish the desired results (Figs 7-3a and 7-3b).

For teeth with existing restorations, you should wait at least 1 month after bleaching before replacing the restoration because of a concern for future marginal integrity. Prerestorative bleaching may reduce bond strength as well as increase marginal leakage of restorations already present.

Before deciding whether to veneer or bleach, carefully examine the patient's enamel, tooth position, and arch form. First look at the enamel shade and structure. How much translucency is present and where is it located? The danger of bleaching translucent enamel is that it may become more translucent, thereby possibly creating the illusion of a darker, rather than lighter, tooth as darkness from the back of the mouth bleeds through. Use the patient's subjective expectation of the finished result as a guide as to whether bleaching alone will suffice. This necessitates understanding their definitions of "white," "bright," and "natural."

before

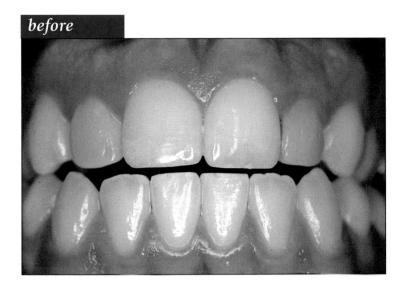

Fig 7-2a Stained composite restorations plus adjacent yellow-brown teeth displease this patient.

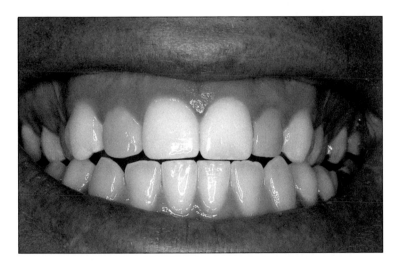

Fig 7-2b A combination of in-office and matrix bleaching treatments lightened the natural teeth but emphasized the darkness of the aging composite-resin restorations.

after

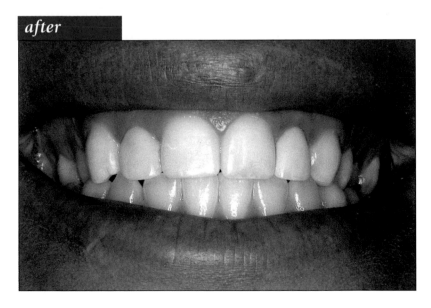

Fig 7-2c Rebonding of the lateral incisors completed this bleaching/bonding smile makeover.

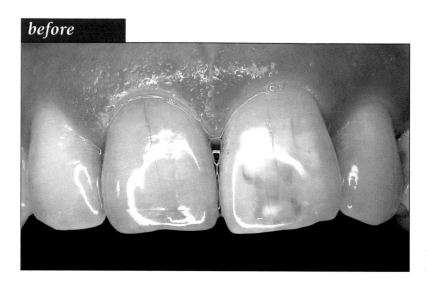

Fig 7-3a Note the brown pigmented areas on the two central incisors.

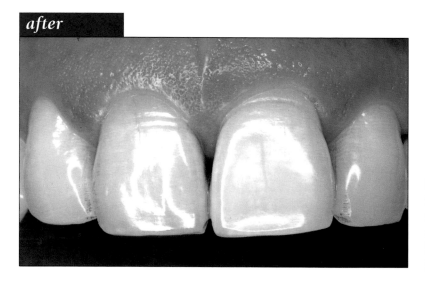

Fig 7-3b In-office external bleaching of the central incisors helped to create a more uniform tooth color. Bonding, laminating, or additional bleaching can always be done should the patient desire a lighter result.

Compromised tooth position or arch arrangement may influence your decision whether to bleach or bond. Although bleaching may well lighten the teeth, the end result may still not please your patient; whiter teeth may still be malpositioned and hence unattractive. Therefore, either bonding or laminating may be a better choice where it is possible to simultaneously create the illusion of straighter teeth. However, the best treatment choice may be orthodontics followed by bleaching, which may produce the best and longest-lasting smile. These choices depend on the patient's personal priorities.

Porcelain Laminate Veneers

When teeth are to be treated with porcelain laminate veneers, the bleaching sequence becomes more critical. With bonding, altering the color is relatively simple if bleaching is not completely effective or varies from the desired shade. This is obviously not possible with porcelain laminates. When the veneer is placed, no color change is possible. In fact, once the technician has completed baking the porcelain, the color is inherent. This means you must make certain the bleached tooth is the desired shade before deciding on the porcelain laminate therapy (Figs 7-4a to 7-4d). Wait at least 3 weeks after the final bleaching session before recording the color.

A more contentious issue is whether or not the patient should continue with home bleaching during the period between making the impressions for the veneers and placing them. Many patients will plead to be allowed to do so, wanting to quickly obtain the lightest possible color change. *Know your patient!* This plan may be fine for a nonperfectionist patient, but a patient who expects precision of color may be disappointed with a less-than-perfect match. And even a perfect match may require ongoing or periodic matrix bleaching, which has been reported by some researchers to affect the porcelain laminates.

> *Wait at least 3 weeks after the final bleaching session before recording the color.*

When lightening both arches, bleaching is a simpler approach to mandibular teeth than trying to laminate this arch. First, it is more difficult technically to laminate mandibular teeth, and both chewing and parafunctional habits tend to cause more failure in this arch. Second, given the natural difference in the amount of lower teeth that show in a smile, bleaching works well. In the typical patient, only a few millimeters of labio-incisal surface of mandibular teeth show during smiling. This incisal third and midportion of the tooth are generally the lightest part of any tooth due to the increased thickness of enamel. In the cervical portion, usually not visible, the discolored dentin below the enamel tends to be more obvious. Third, bleaching works very well on the visible part of lower teeth because the incisal portion, being largely enamel, absorbs more of the bleaching solution.

before

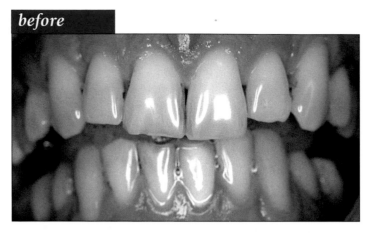

Fig 7-4a This 41-year-old man was dissatisfied with his discolored teeth.

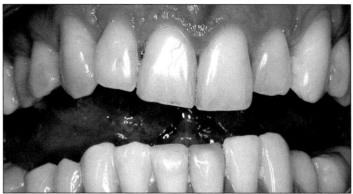

Fig 7-4b The mandibular teeth were bleached first, using the maxillary teeth as a control. Note arch irregularity caused partially by tooth wear and subsequent eruption.

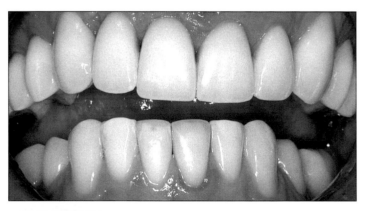

Fig 7-4c Initial bleaching of the mandibular teeth allowed the use of lighter-colored porcelain laminates for the maxillary teeth.

after

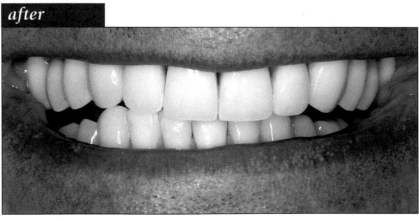

Fig 7-4d The final smile shows not only lighter color, but also improved arch symmetry through 12 porcelain laminates on the maxillary teeth.

Finally, the upper and lower teeth do not have to match perfectly, since the two arches are rarely seen adjacent to each other and the lower teeth are usually lingually placed, creating a natural shadow behind the maxillary areas.

With bleaching and laminates, as with bonding, it is crucial to understand the satisfaction level of each patient. You can explain all of the above issues, but if your patient is a perfectionist, a full set of identically colored upper and lower laminates may be the treatment of choice.

Crowns

In certain situations, crowns remain the treatment of choice because of their strength or the need to splint several restorative units. Cosmetically, crowns can neutralize underlying darkly stained teeth and be lightened or matched to any shade. Often, teeth that were originally restored before the advent of composite-resin bonding or porcelain-laminate veneers need to be recrowned. In any such scenario, if the adjacent and/or opposing teeth are to be lightened, bleaching must be performed first for two reasons. First, it is extremely difficult to bleach adjacent teeth to match a crown, but crown fabrication can match the tooth color achieved during bleaching. Second, exposure of the new crown and cementing medium to bleaching solution should be minimized (Figs 7-5a to 7-5d).

Wait at least 2 to 3 weeks following the last bleaching treatment to select the shade for matching the crowns. Be forewarned that many patients will be resistant to this delay and will ask you to proceed to crown the tooth using a lighter shade than ultimately indicated. To do this is potentially problematic, as such requests are based on a common misconception among patients that bleaching can be done incrementally, stopping when the shade is pleasing. If the patient insists, a preferable approach is to speed up the bleaching process with two sessions of in-office power bleaching, followed by use of a matrix while the crown is being fabricated. This will give you a better sense of the ultimate shade possible with bleaching. Carefully review the treatment plan, especially the limitations of bleaching, with the patient!

before

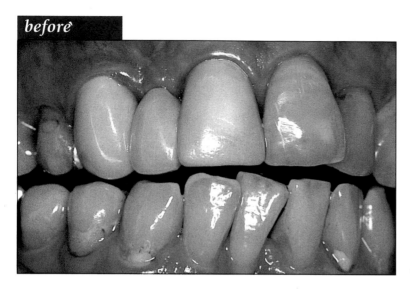

Fig 7-5a This 63-year-old woman was unhappy with her crooked and discolored teeth.

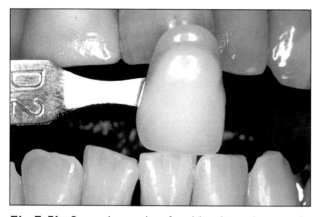

Fig 7-5b Several months after bleaching the mandibular teeth, the final shade was recorded for the maxillary restorative treatment.

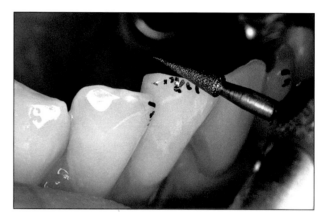

Fig 7-5c The mandibular teeth were also cosmetically contoured to make them appear straighter.

after

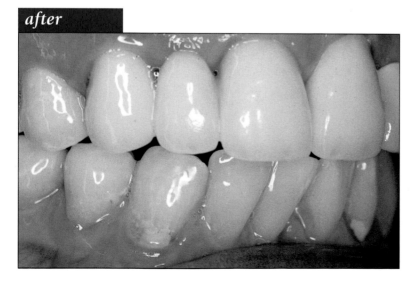

Fig 7-5d The maxillary prosthesis can be fabricated in a slightly lighter shade than that of the bleached mandibular anterior teeth.

Bleaching in Conjunction with Periodontal Care

Many of your patients will be under the care of a periodontist or will need to have one included as part of their overall treatment plan. Periodontal disease is one of the most common health problems in this country, supposedly affecting 95% of all adults at some time during their life. It also is a major cause of changes in adult smiles, the leading cause of adult tooth loss, receding gums, loss of interdental space, and changes in lip-line relationship.

As a general rule, bleaching follows oral disease control and treatment of any periodontal disease. If there is evidence of inflammatory periodontal disease, this must be corrected before any bleaching is undertaken. If periodontal problems have created gingival hyperplasia that covers enamel, bleaching must be postponed until after the periodontal surgery exposes the entire crown. If this is not done, a color differential may result in the subgingival unbleached portion in a patient subsequently treated surgically.

Gingival Recession

When recession of gingival tissue has left a void and an unattractive loss of interdental tissues, you may contemplate using pink or tooth-colored composite resin to bond the teeth and fill in the interdental spaces. In this case, periodontal treatment is the primary procedure, followed by bleaching, and finally bonding. This will ensure a better match with the lighter tooth color.

Gingival recession associated with clefting should be evaluated by a periodontist to determine if periodontal surgery can repair and possibly replace the lost tissue. This decision should also be made before any bleaching is attempted.

In patients with advanced bone loss, considerable cementum may be exposed, requiring eventual restoration with bonding, lamination, or crowning. To bleach these teeth before laminating or crowning is a waste of your time and the patient's money. However, if cervical bonding is selected as the treatment of choice, then bleaching is best done in advance. Be sure to place the rubber dam or rubber dam substitute (Den Mat or Ultradent) over the cementum area that will eventually be covered with composite resin (see Fig 3-4).

before

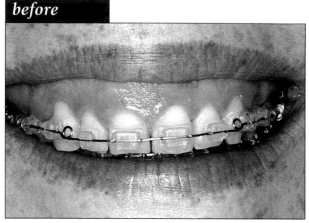

Fig 7-6a Following orthodontics, the patient had well-aligned teeth but disharmony between their position and the inferior border of the upper lip. This "gummy" smile is the result of vertical maxillary excess.

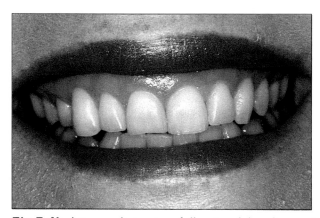

Fig 7-6b Intermediate view following debanding and orthognathic surgery, which involved vertical impaction of the maxilla.

after

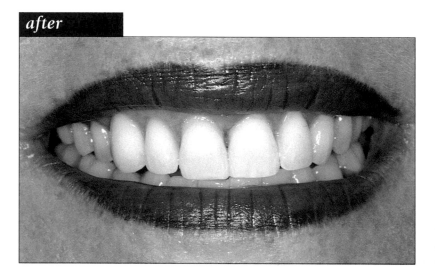

Fig 7-6c Final result showing total dentofacial harmony, developed using surgical procedures, orthodontics, cosmetic contouring, and bleaching.

If periodontal care precedes bleaching, wait at least 6 to 12 weeks after surgery before bleaching, since placement of the rubber dam may irritate the gum tissue.

Only when the planned periodontal therapy or surgery will not alter the amount of tooth surface to be bleached and any inflammation is under control may bleaching precede periodontal treatment. Such cases would include patients whose tissues have already receded or those whose lip lines are so low that periodontal surgery will have no effect on the amount of tooth exposed *during smiling*.

Bleaching in Conjunction with Orthodontic Care

Orthodontic treatment is utilized to improve esthetics, function, and phonetics for patients. For many years, orthodontics was used only in children and adolescents, but today more than 40% of all orthodontic patients are adults. The importance of teamwork and mutual understanding between the orthodontist and the dentist performing bleaching and other esthetic procedures cannot be overemphasized.

The sequence of orthodontics and bleaching depends on which of the following four general categories applies to the patient:

1. When major orthodontic correction involving fixed appliances is indicated, it is preferable to wait until the appliances are removed and any remaining cement or bonded resin material is thoroughly cleaned from the teeth. Obviously, little, if any, effective bleaching can be performed while the patient is wearing fixed appliances. For most patients, waiting is not a problem and bleaching is seen as the next logical step following orthodontics.

2. For some patients, enhanced esthetics in any form is of paramount importance and initial lightening of darkened teeth will suffice. In this case, it may be desirable to bleach the teeth before the ceramic or metal brackets are bonded to them, scheduling bleaching treatments in conjunction with the orthodontist.

3. When minor therapy with removable appliances is underway, bleaching can be done simultaneously (Figs 7-7a to 7-7e). It is important to know if a tooth is going to be moved slightly or an arch realigned or expanded, however, since it may be easier to bleach specific teeth before placing an appliance.

4. The combined matrix technique developed by Goldstein and Salama raises new possibilities for collaboration between orthodontists and the general dentist (Figs 7-8a to 7-8c). Working much like a repositioning appliance to move teeth into a more appropriate position and retain them there, the matrix can be made to hold a mild bleaching solution as well. Make sure air-vent holes are placed between the arches so the bleaching solution does not leak out. Our initial experience has been that home bleaching serves as a more immediate patient reinforcement to wearing the matrix during sleep or while at home. If long-range

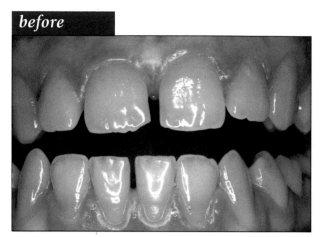

Fig 7-7a This 19-year-old woman was concerned about her discolored and malpositioned teeth.

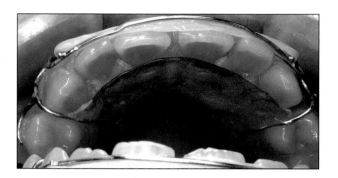

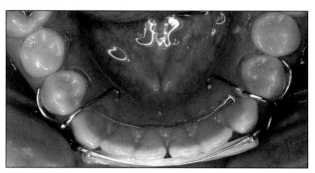

Fig 7-7b and 7-7c Removable Hawley-type appliances were constructed to close the spaces. Elastics were also used to help accelerate tooth movement.

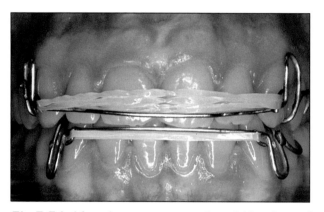

Fig 7-7d After the spaces were closed, bleaching of the maxillary teeth was started during the retention phase of treatment.

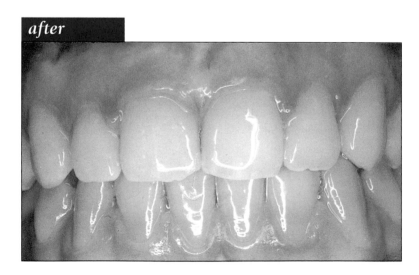

Fig 7-7e By the time the teeth were retained (approximately 3 months), in-office bleaching treatments helped achieve the improved tooth color.

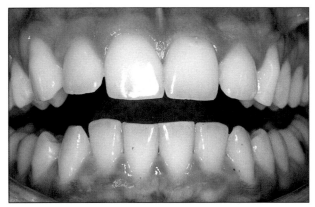

Fig 7-8a This patient has mild anterior crowding to be improved with an orthodontic repositioning appliance.

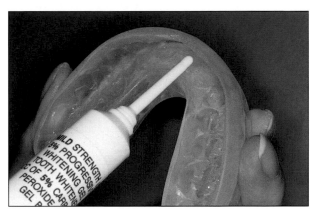

Fig 7-8b Since the patient wanted her teeth lighter as well as straighter, the repositioner will serve also as a bleaching matrix. The bleaching gel is being placed as directed.

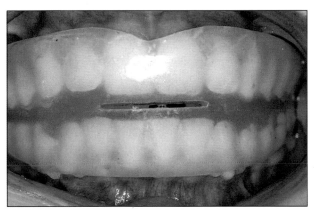

Fig 7-8c Combined matrix/retainer for patient wear, which will accomplish bleaching at the same time the teeth are being straightened.

studies support these initial findings, many orthodontists may be grateful for a solution to the common problem of retainers spending the night in a drawer instead of their user's mouth.

Bleaching in Conjunction with Other Esthetic Treatments

While bleaching won't solve every problem, it can often be a significant and effective preparatory or adjunctive treatment. The patient must fully understand bleaching's limitations and remember that any teeth with metallic restorations that influence the tooth color should have those restorations removed before bleaching. This is also true when making any shade decisions prior to bonding or veneering. Replacement restorations may be composite resin or ceramic (Figs 7-9a to 7-9d).

Cosmetic Contouring

The two most common traits of "attractive" smiles are usually "straight" and "white." These two qualities can often be achieved through the combined conservative efforts of cosmetic contouring and bleaching teeth. Cosmetic contouring, or reshaping natural teeth to achieve an illusion of straightness, can be done to some extent on almost every patient. Goldstein reported in 1987 that in one study of individuals considered attractive, over 95% of those surveyed could have had some improvement through cosmetic contouring. Almost everyone can have a more attractive smile through reshaping teeth to improve silhouette form. The easiest way to see silhouette form is through a photograph or video image, because they create a two-dimensional view, rather than a three-dimensional view. The vertical or horizontal overlaps can be contoured provided occlusion is stable. Simring reported that either centric or protrusive contacts can be altered, provided one or the other remains intact, and still retains stability of the occlusion.

Although the order in which the procedures are accomplished is not critical, bleaching is generally done first so that once the teeth are lighter, cosmetic contouring brings about the desired esthetic transformation. It is not uncommon after completing both bleaching and cosmetic contouring for patients to question

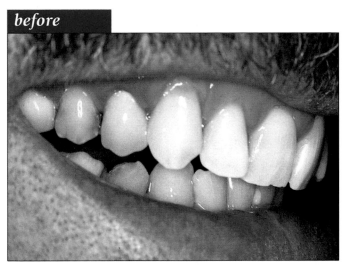

before

Fig 7-9a This patient was dissatisfied with his discolored teeth.

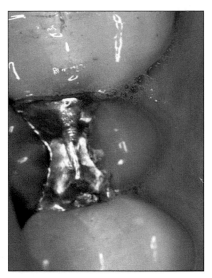

Fig 7-9b Note the defective amalgam restoration that made the discoloration more noticeable.

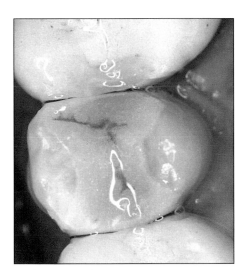

Fig 7-9c Before bleaching was attempted, the amalgam restoration was replaced with a porcelain inlay.

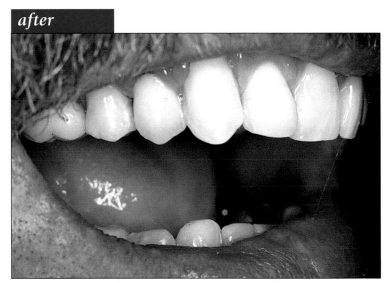

after

Fig 7-9d The combined effect of replacing the restoration plus bleaching provided a much lighter and more attractive smile.

whether or not additional restorative therapy is necessary. If the patient is happy with this initial therapy, then certainly the conservative approach of not subjecting patients to the more invasive procedures of bonded, laminated or crowned restorations (with their decreased lifespans and need for ongoing retreatment) is advantageous—if the patient is happy!

In integrated therapy, the combination of cosmetic contouring and bleaching is incorporated into most other restorative treatments to achieve as harmonious a smile as possible. Therefore, it is important during treatment planning to use a checklist listing all of the various options, so that each treatment can be considered in your diagnostic decision and treatment planning (Figs 7-10a to 7-10c).

Abrasive Techniques

Abrasive techniques are sometimes used before bleaching to remove deep stains or to minimize white or brown spots. While bleaching alone will not usually remove these spots, there are three approaches that may make bleaching an appropriate follow-up or combined treatment. These approaches are diamond-stone surface alteration, chemical-physical microabrasion, and kinetic-energy preparation (abrasive technology).

Both microabrasion and abrasive technology can be thought of as a form of controlled color enhancement through enamel removal. The Prema (Premier Dental Products) compound contains abrasive particles suspended with a low concentration of hydrochloric acid in a water-soluble gel. It is applied to enamel with a hard rubber mandrel in a low-speed handpiece at 20- to 30-second intervals for 5 to 10 minutes, depending upon the depth of the stain, followed by enamel surface polishing with a rubber cup and fine-grit fluoridated prophy paste. Microabrasion actually removes 22 to 27 μm of the enamel per application by softening the enamel with hydrochloric acid and abrading it with a controlled abrasive technique (Figs 7-11a to 7-11f). The KCP2000 (American Dental Technology) uses two sizes of abrasive powder particles under high pressure to erode away enamel defects. This more controlled process conservatively takes out stains or white spots (or even caries, occasionally leaving a defect which then can be easily filled with composite resin).

before

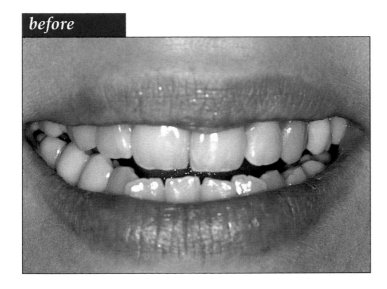

Fig 7-10a This patient was unhappy with her discolored and crowded teeth.

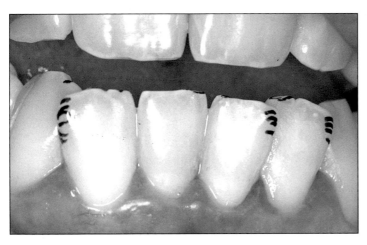

Fig 7-10b An alcohol marker (Masel Orthodontics) is used to mark the teeth to be both repositioned and contoured.

after

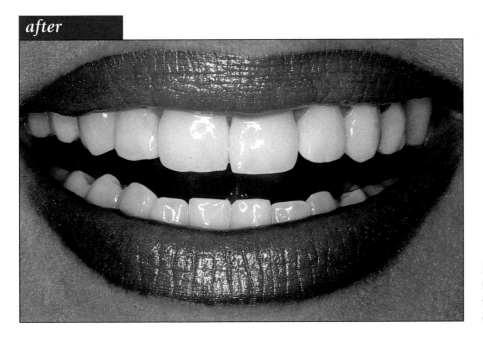

Fig 7-10c Orthodontics, bleaching, and cosmetic contouring were combined to create the final result.

before

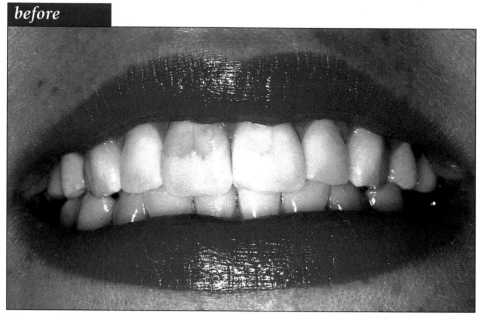

Fig 7-11a Yellow-brown staining on the central incisors. Microabrasion combined with bleaching was chosen as the treatment of choice.

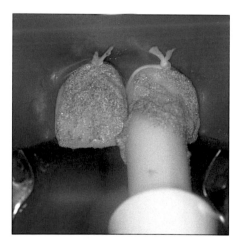

Fig 7-11b After placement of the rubber dam, the abrasive compound (Prema, Premier) was applied under pressure with a hand applicator using a rubbing motion.

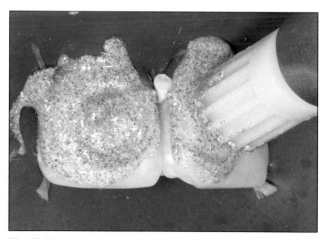

Fig 7-11c A rotary instrument attached to a special gear-reduction contra-angle handpiece was used for 20- to 30-second intervals for approximately 5 to 10 minutes to polish and remove the stain.

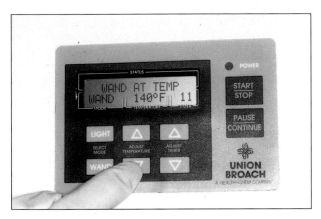

Fig 7-11d A bleaching wand (Illuminator, Union Broach) with programmable temperature was used to individually bleach the two central incisors following microabrasion treatment.

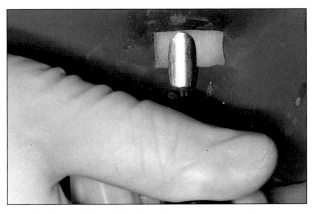

Fig 7-11e When the bleaching wand reached the preprogrammed temperature, it was applied to the 35% hydrogen peroxide–saturated gauze intermittently for approximately 5 minutes.

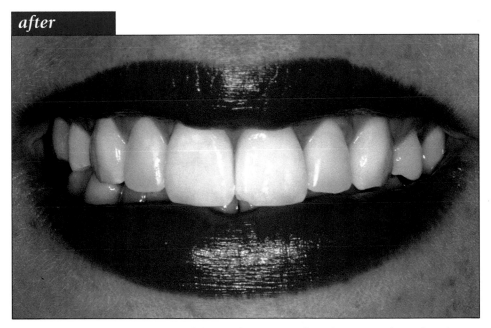

Fig 7-11f Three applications of this technique produced improved tooth color.

Microabrasion or use of the KCP2000 for white spots provides an excellent illustration of how bleaching can serve as a first step that may prove to be sufficient for the patient, thus saving further treatment, or that may improve the existing situation for the next step in smile enhancement.

For many patients, the ultimate restoration may appear to be laminates because they can closely match the color of other teeth and provide needed correction for tooth form and arrangement. The patient, however, may prefer a less invasive and, more often, a less costly approach. In this case, you may suggest trying the more conservative alternative, knowing veneers can still be used if necessary. Use the guidelines in Chapter 3 for providing information and documenting the patient's acceptance of your assessment of the diminished likelihood of success using bleaching as an alternative treatment.

The final result may be satisfactory, especially to a patient with a low esthetic "satisfaction quotient" (see page 55). When it is not satisfactory, the bleaching will have neutralized the tooth color somewhat and have served as a useful step toward the more appropriate treatment.

Combining Bleaching with Orthognathic or Plastic Surgery

In these situations, bleach before the surgery, especially if in-office bleaching is to be used. Patients who plan to have plastic surgery or orthognathic surgery are frequently concerned that the application of the rubber dam will cause stretching of the tissue. In our practice, we have had patients express mental anguish because their cheeks were being "puffed out" by the placement of cotton rolls during treatment. If the patient already has had the surgical treatment, it is advisable to select matrix bleaching to minimize patient concerns about stretching and to protect yourself from complaints, and perhaps even legal action, the first time the patient sees a facial wrinkle.

Bibliography

Anderson M. Dental bleaching. Curr Sci 1991;1:185–191.

Crim G. Prerestorative bleaching: Effect on microleakage of class V cavities. Quintessence Int 1992;23:823–825.

Dzierzak J. Factors which cause tooth color changes . . . protocol for in-office power bleaching. Pract Periodont Aesthet Dent 1991;3(2):15–20.

Friedman M. Conservative management of discolored dentition. GP 1992;Mar:45–48.

Goldstein RE. Bleaching teeth: New materials–new role. J Am Dent Assoc 1987, Dec (special issue):44E–52E.

Goldstein RE. Study of need for esthetics in dentistry. J Prosthet Dent 1969;21(6):589–598.

Goldstein RE. Dentists note concerns and advice about vital tooth bleaching (interview). Gen Dent 1990;Jan/Feb:8–11.

Goldstein RE, Salama MA. Integrated orthodontic and bleaching therapy, in press.

Haywood V, Williams H. Stains and restorative options for dentist prescribed home-applied bleaching. Esthetic Dent Update 1994; 5(3):65–67.

Killian C. Conservative color improvement. J Am Dent Assoc 1993; 124(May):72–74.

Magne P, Magne M, Belser U. Natural and restorative oral esthetics. Part 2: Esthetic treatment modalities. JEsthet Dent 1993;5(6):239–246.

McEvoy S. Chemical agents for removing intrinsic stains from vital teeth: Technique development. Quintessence Int 1989;20:323–327.

Rada RE. Safe and effective vital tooth bleaching. CDS Rev, Sept, 1993.

Simring M. Practical periodontal techniques for esthetics. Postgraduate course. First Dist Dent Soc of NY. November 1966.

Weinstein A. Bleaching, bonding and veneering: A rationale for material and technique choice. Aesthet Chron 1992;3(4):34–41.

Index

Numbers in *italic* refer to pages in which figures appear